The Juice Lady's Turbo Diet

Cherie Calbom

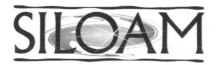

Most CHARISMA HOUSE BOOK GROUP products are available at special quantity discounts for bulk purchase for sales promotions, premiums, fund-raising, and educational needs. For details, write Charisma House Book Group, 600 Rinehart Road, Lake Mary, Florida 32746, or telephone (407) 333-0600.

THE JUICE LADY'S TURBO DIET by Cherie Calbom
Published by Siloam, Charisma Media/Charisma House Book Group
600 Rinehart Road, Lake Mary, Florida 32746
www.charismahouse.com

Cover design by Bill Johnson
Cherie's photograph by Marianne Lyle

Copyright © 2010 by Cherie Calbom
All rights reserved

Library of Congress Cataloging-in-Publication Data
Calbom, Cherie.
　The juice lady's turbo diet / Cherie Calbom. -- 1st ed.
　　p. cm.
　Includes bibliographical references and index.
　ISBN 978-1-61638-149-3
　1. Reducing diets. 2. Fruit juices. 3. Vegetable juices. 4.
Detoxification (Health). 5. Reducing diets--Recipes. I. Title.
　RM222.2.C227 2010
　613.2'6--dc22
　　　　　　　　　　　　　2010006042

This book contains the opinions and ideas of its author. It is solely for informational and educational purposes and should not be regarded as a substitute for professional medical treatment. The nature of your body's health condition is complex and unique. Therefore you should consult a health professional before you begin any new exercise, nutrition, or supplementation program or if you have questions about your health. Neither the author nor the publisher shall be liable or responsible for any loss or damage allegedly arising from any information or suggestion in this book.

Names and details of testimonials of some individuals mentioned in this book have been changed, and any similarity between the names and stories of individuals described in this book to individuals known to readers is purely coincidental.

The statements in this book about consumable products or food have not been evaluated by the Food and Drug Administration. The recipes in this book are to be followed exactly as written. Neither the publisher nor the author is responsible for your specific health or allergy needs that may require medical supervision. The publisher and the author are not responsible for any adverse reactions to the consumption of food or products that have been suggested in this book.

While the author has made every effort to provide accurate telephone numbers and Internet addresses at the time of publication, neither the publisher nor the author assumes any responsibility for errors or for changes that occur after publication.

E-book ISBN: 978-1-61638-246-9

11 12 13 14 — 9 8 7 6 5 4
Printed in the United States of America

To Abba, the Source of all life

Acknowledgments

To those who have assisted us with this book, I am forever grateful.

- To my editor, Debbie Marrie: You're the best! You've added such valuable input to this book.
- To my literary agent, Pamela Harty: Once again you helped me find a home for my work.
- I also wish to express my deep and lasting appreciation to all the other people who have helped to make *The Juice Lady's Turbo Diet* a success.
- Lastly, I want to thank the Holy Trinity and the angels who have assisted me in writing this book. To my dear heavenly Father, Jesus Christ, and Holy Spirit, thank You for guiding me throughout this project. You showed me Your ways of wisdom, creativity, and truth as to how to care for the human body. You've guided me to the fountain of life in the juicing and cleansing programs I've been able to develop. Thank You for the health I've come to enjoy. I also thank You for the awesome responsibility of helping other people lose weight and discover a way of life that truly promotes health. For the blessings You've given me and Your unconditional love, I am so very grateful.

Contents

Foreword

Two out of three people in the United States struggle with obesity. This is a relatively modern trend, and it is likely related to recent innovations in food processing that have diverted us away from natural, healthy, unprocessed foods.

Probably the largest culprit is the massive increase in consumption of fructose, which is now the number one source of calories in the United States. It is no mystery that sugar is not good for you, but fructose is particularly pernicious.

Most fructose is metabolized directly to fat—unlike glucose, which is more typically converted to energy. Additionally, fructose will massively increase insulin and leptin resistance, which are primary foundational causes of inability to lose weight.

The wonderful aspect of Cherie's approach is that she provides you with a very low fructose diet that tends to normalize most of the complex biochemistry associated with consuming fructose in excess of 15 grams per day.

Not only is fructose limited by this approach, but it is also replaced with some of the most essential foods that you could possibly consume. They are loaded with micronutrients and biophotons that are virtually impossible to obtain in any dietary supplement.

Juicing can be an important part of a successful weight loss program because most of us have impaired digestion as a result of making less-than-optimal food choices. This can limit your body's ability to absorb all the nutrients from vegetables. Juicing will help to "predigest" them for you, so you will receive most of the nutrients.

Juicing helps you absorb all the nutrients from the vegetables and can help you add a far larger variety of vegetables than you would normally consume in your diet.

Many people eat the same vegetable salads every day. This violates the principle of eating a large variety of foods and actually increases your chance of developing food allergies. Juicing allows you to consume a wide variety of vegetables that you may not normally enjoy eating whole.

The majority of people are pleasantly surprised to find that juicing is much easier than they thought it would be. Ideally, you should start juicing vegetables that you enjoy eating whole and fresh.

If you have had challenges losing weight, you owe it to yourself to try this approach. The odds are overwhelming that it will help you with your efforts. You will also be healthier, and you will radically reduce your risk for developing chronic degenerative diseases as you get older.

—DR. JOSEPH MERCOLA
FOUNDER, MERCOLA.COM—WORLD'S MOST VISITED
NATURAL HEALTH SITE

Introduction

Y OU MAY HAVE tried nearly every diet on the planet. Have you choked down more grapefruit than you ever want to see again? Perhaps you've purchased boxes and boxes of diet food. What else? Flushed the fat? Eaten no fat or low fat? Maybe you've polished off enough protein to support an animal feed lot. But alas, as the song goes, *you're right back where you started from.* Well, hold your chin up! You will never need to go looking for another diet again if you follow *The Juice Lady's Turbo Diet.* It's a healthy, easy, antiaging, disease-preventing diet. Best of all—it works!

I'll let you in on a secret. The Turbo Diet really isn't a diet. *It's a way of life!* It's a plan you can follow year after year until you say *au revoir* to this life. It's the way of eating that I've followed for more than two decades. I know it works. It's how I've maintained my weight. It's worked for hundreds of people that I've worked with as a nutritionist and the Juice Lady.

I became the Juice Lady in 1991 when I went to work for the Juiceman Company while I was finishing my master of science degree at Bastyr University. Since graduating in 1991, I've spoken to audiences, both large and small, at halls, restaurants, meeting rooms, convention centers, churches, and universities. I've taught cooking, juicing, nutrition, and weight-loss classes for many years. Hundreds of people have lost weight and improved their health by applying what they've learned in my classes and groups. The juicing program has been proven to facilitate weight loss in university studies, which you'll read more about in chapter 1. Now you can enjoy the weight-loss benefits of the Turbo Diet along with abundant energy, better mood, and improved health.

The Turbo Diet revolution kicked off with the May 4, 2009, issue of *Woman's World* magazine's cover story "The Turbo Juice Diet." Cover girl Sarah Taylor lost 20 pounds on this diet and landed on the cover of the magazine. She had attended one of my juicing and cleansing classes

1

in the Seattle area. She bought a juicer and headed home to try juicing to see what would happen. But she didn't use my juice recipe book *The Juice Lady's Guide to Juicing for Health*. Rather, she bought a bunch of produce including a gingerroot and juiced the whole thing. It tasted so bad she decided never to try *that* again—that was until her friend Channah lost 13 pounds for her wedding on the juicing program. Not only did Channah look fabulously trim, but also her skin was clear and glowing. She had more energy than before. And she was sold on juicing for life. So Sarah decided she'd try again—this time with some of my recipes. They tasted great! She continued juicing, and the weight just melted away. You can read more of her story on page 8.

Losing weight is not just about getting rid of fat; it's about getting to the cause of why you gained weight in the first place. The Turbo Diet is all about helping you discover the source of your weight gain and teaching you how to enjoy a diet and lifestyle that keeps weight off for good. This diet gets to the root of the choices that contributed to your weight gain in the first place. It's like spreading landscape fabric to prevent weeds from growing rather than pulling up weeds all the time. When you understand what sets you up for weight gain, you will understand how to stay trim and fit.

Here's why the Turbo Diet works so well. It changes your internal landscape so not only will you get trim, but you will also gain energy and get healthier. Nearly everyone, like Sarah, has said that weight loss became a secondary gain to all the other health benefits of this diet. It's a plan that serves up freshly made veggie juices twice a day with delicious high-alkaline, low-glycemic foods that help you melt away fat and keep it off for good! This simple program details exactly how you can reach your ideal weight. It works so well because it feeds the body an abundance of vitamins, minerals, enzymes, and phytonutrients in the form of freshly made juices and high-water content, alkaline plant foods like vegetables, low-sugar fruit, and sprouts. To that you add small portions of lean protein, seeds, nuts, and whole grains, and you have the diet for success.

And listen up! This is a proven program. It is based on scientific studies that you will learn more about as you read on, which confirm that drinking two glasses of veggie juice daily increased weight loss four times over those who drank no juice.

One definition of *turbo* is "to increase the power of." The fresh, raw vegetable juices recommended in this program can increase the power of a high-alkaline, low-glycemic diet and have the potential to make it a turbo-charged recipe for success.

With this diet you will have a chance to truly feed your body. When you are satisfied nutritionally, your cravings fade away like mist before the sun. Your body can use everything you eat. Very little gets stored up in fat cells. A lot of those little "storage tanks" won't be needed much longer.

This program doesn't contribute to a buildup of acid or toxins in your body either. Therefore, your system won't need to shuttle off a bunch of harmful stuff into fat cells and hold on to them "for dear life." Voilà! You're losing weight while hardly trying.

Chock-full of nutrients, the vegetable juice combinations in the Turbo Diet, along with the delicious food recipes, send a signal to the brain that your body is well fed. You will be less likely to experience hunger signals that cause you to clean out the fridge after dinner because your body is still starving for nutrients. And because the juices are rich in antioxidants that bind to toxins and carry them off, they help detoxify the stuff that is a major source of weight gain— toxins and acids. Not only have many people lost weight on the Turbo Diet, but they've also soon discovered it's a lifestyle they want to keep because they feel so great—like having abundant energy, better sleep, and a happier state of mind. There are many testimonies attesting to these benefits within the pages of this book, and more stories on my Web site www.juiceladyinfo.com.

But there's more. How about getting rid of cellulite? You will find out why this diet works to rid your body of that lumpy skin that looks like an orange peel. And how about improving sugar imbalances like hypoglycemia, insulin resistance, or diabetes? You will learn why this program helps balance blood sugar and correct insulin resistance. And it doesn't end there. Throughout these pages, you will discover the many ways the Turbo Diet can help you improve your health.

Most people who embark on the Turbo Diet report exciting benefits that reach far beyond weight loss. In fact, loads of "happy losers" have said that the energy and good health they've experienced were more important to them than the weight they dropped. "I'm waking up happy most mornings, which is a first," said Karen, "and my family likes to be around me." She's not alone. Nita reported that not only did she lose 42 pounds, but also her hot flashes in the night are completely gone. Francine, who has lost 54 pounds, said she gained so much energy she took up ballroom dancing and actually entered some competitions. What would you like to accomplish or enjoy?

THE JUICE DIET THAT WORKS!

With a fourteen-day varied meal plan and scores of scrumptious recipes, you're on your way to a new you! You can enjoy many delicious foods and a variety of vegetable juices while melting away fat. That's all you have to do. Just think; you can eat great-tasting food, drink delicious vegetable juices, and lose weight!

The Juice Lady's Turbo Diet is fun, easy, and healthy. It gets results without struggle or deprivation—without cravings or climbing the kitchen wall. You will feel satisfied after drinking the fresh vegetable juices. And you will be smiling when you step on the bathroom scale.

Seven Reasons Why the Turbo Diet Works

1. It supplies an abundance of nutrients that satisfy the body. Cravings usually diminish quickly.

2. It feeds the brain supernutrients that send a signal to the body that it's satisfied. People often say they aren't hungry after a big glass of fresh veggie juice.

3. Live juices detoxify the body. Toxins can actually cause us to gain weight. It's true. And they can make it very difficult to lose fat.

4. The Turbo Diet is energizing. For a majority of people, fatigue vanishes and workouts get easier. When you work out, you build muscle and burn calories. The more muscle you develop, the more calories you burn, even when resting.

5. It's low in calories. If you're counting them, this program is low in those little energy units that push up the numbers on the bathroom scale.

6. It is low glycemic, meaning it's devoid of fattening carbs.

7. It's a high-alkaline diet. This is a major factor to consider. Actually, the body stores acids in fat cells to protect delicate tissues and organs, making it tough to get rid of fat when the diet is predominantly acidic. Listen up–the body will actually make fat to store acids when it runs out of storage space. When you achieve a healthy pH balance, your body can start letting go of fat cells.

A New Way of Life

When you complete the Turbo Diet, my hope is that you will have changed your internal chemistry and established new eating habits. The cravings and urges that once lured you to snack foods you didn't even want should be gone. If emotional eating and binge eating trip you up, chapter 6 has scores of ideas to help you conquer those inner triggers. Yo-yo dieting could be gone forever—if you make this style of eating your way of life.

Best of all—you will be healthier. Just as in the success stories people share with me daily through letters and e-mails, you too may experience more weight-loss success, coupled with energy and abundant health, than you have ever thought possible. You can have a happier mood and the opportunity to enjoy each day. And you will stand the greatest chance of preventing serious diseases like cancer, diabetes, or heart disease.

If you reach a roadblock, chapter 5's troubleshooting tips should help you correct some underlying issues that have been keeping you from reaching your goals. Just think how grateful you will be when you have corrected some health problems that had you stymied and discouraged.

This is the diet you will want to stick with because feeling healthy, happy, and energetic is something you will never want to lose once you attain it—no matter how alluring some foods might be. So lift your glass of veggie juice and toast to a new era in your life!

Chapter 1

The Turbo Diet

I ANSWERED THE PHONE one afternoon to hear the excited voice of Denise at the other end of the line. She had just lost 8 pounds on the Turbo Diet. Having read about it in the cover story of *Woman's World* magazine's May 4, 2009, issue, she had tried the juice diet as a last resort. "It's just amazing to me," she said, "that I've lost this much weight so quickly and easily. I've dieted and dieted on all sorts of plans and couldn't lose any weight. I even went on a strict three-day water fast and hardly lost anything. Now, the weight is just melting off. It's amazing!"

Amazing is a word I hear frequently about this diet.

Why have so many people found the Turbo Diet to be amazing? Simply said—it works!

The Turbo Diet is loaded with nutrients—enzymes, minerals, vitamins, phytonutrients, and life! That's right! It's full of those little energy sparks we call *life*. Fresh raw juices are considered live food because they feed the body a cornucopia of nutrients that have not been destroyed by heat or processing along with the energy the plants absorb from the sun. This diet is also high alkaline, low acidic, and low glycemic. Achieving a healthy alkaline-acid balance through your diet and lifestyle is so important to weight loss and health that once you understand the importance of this factor, vegetable juices will taste even better.

On the Turbo Diet, "the munchies" just seem to disappear. You might realize one day that you don't want the junk food you used to eat. In fact, you will probably find that junk food makes you feel awful and it's just not worth it. I'm not saying that a potato chip won't ever lure you into its grip. But you will be better able to resist the call of that starch, grease, and salt when your body is well fed and pulsating with energy.

Freshly made vegetable juices are at the center of the Turbo Diet. They provide concentrated sources of very absorbable nutrients. They are low in fat and calories, so replacing higher-calorie foods with fresh juice is a shoo-in for weight-loss success.

But the benefits of juicing don't stop there. Vegetable juices help curb cravings because they satisfy your body's nutrient needs. They're alkaline, which is very helpful to balance out a system that's probably too acidic. They're also high in antioxidants that are antiaging and immune enhancing—that means you're giving your body the things it needs to start looking and feeling younger. How cool is that!

And this diet doesn't toss the carrots out with the potato chips because all carbohydrates are not created equal. You will learn which carbohydrates are healthy and which are not as you discover why the low-glycemic diet works so well with vegetable juices. Your taste buds will be happy—*the juices taste great!* But clearly the most important aspect is that juicing helps you improve your health. And since you get one precious body for one lifetime, that's far more important than just getting skinny.

The Juice Lady's Turbo Diet teaches you how to eat healthily to stay trim by consuming good carbohydrates, lean proteins (unless you're vegan), healthy fats, and two glasses of fresh vegetable juice each day. You will be arming your body with an arsenal of powerful weapons to help you lose weight, lose cravings, and get healthy—maybe healthier than you have been in years. That's weight loss with a mission!

Sarah Lost 20 Pounds and Landed on the Cover of *Woman's World*!

Radio broadcaster Sarah Taylor was on the cover of the May 4, 2009, issue of *Woman's World* magazine and the featured person in the Turbo Juice Diet story. "I'm currently down 20 pounds, which is HUGE for me, as I haven't successfully lost weight in years," said Sarah. "But the best part is that I wasn't trying to lose weight. I just incorporated healthy, live foods through juicing for nutrition. The weight loss was just a bonus!" She said she started filling herself up with the right foods and her body said thank you! "I lost 20 pounds in ten weeks," she added. "This is the only diet that's ever worked for me. I love it!"

The Secrets of the Turbo Diet

Vegetable juice is the secret ingredient to your weight-loss success. It assists you in becoming slim and healthy due to its alkalinizing, nutrition-packed, energizing properties. Let's face it—juicing is a lot easier than spending all your time chowing down brussels sprouts, carrots, and broccoli. Don't get me wrong. I recommend that you eat these vegetables often, but really, just how many vegetables can you eat in a day? But you can juice them and drink them with ease.

Because vegetable juice has very little sugar, while offering an abundance of vitamins, minerals, enzymes, and phytonutrients, it's incredibly helpful for weight loss. It offers what your body needs to fight cravings and do its work to keep you healthy. You will not only want to eat fewer calories when you include vegetable juicing in your daily routine, but you will also gain energy. On the other hand, you can eat a whole bag of chips and still want something more to eat because your body was given a lot of empty calories that made you feel sluggish and tired. The biggest plus of a juicing program is that it adds valuable nutrients (vitamins, minerals, enzymes, and phytonutrients) that are easy for your body to absorb and that have a heap of health benefits at minimal calorie cost.

You will be downing highly concentrated health cocktails brimming with life and loaded with nature's bounty of nutrition necessary for vitality and a healthy immune system. This facilitates optimal functioning of all your body's systems.

Most of us are very aware of the side effects of unhealthy appetite suppressants or risky surgery, but sometimes people feel that they have no other option. I'm here to tell you that you *do* have options, and the Turbo Diet is one of the healthiest options on the earth! The vegetable juices act as healthy, harmless appetite suppressants. You can opt for a glass of fresh veggie juice before your main meal and quickly experience those hunger pangs taking an exit. That's just one of the secret reasons why the Turbo Diet works.

Dave the Trucker Lost Over 230 Pounds by Juicing!

Sometimes people say that they just don't have time to juice. My answer is that there's always time and creative ways to accomplish what we value. I have a friend known as "Dave the 'Raw Foods' Trucker" who's lost a *truckload* of weight by juicing. Dave was desperate to drop about half his weight and restore his health. Weighing in at 430 pounds, he faced losing his job because of his poor health. He had no idea how he would earn a living if he lost his driving profession. To say the least, this made him anxious to find an answer that worked quickly.

When a friend introduced him to vegetable juicing, it made sense that this could change his life. Dave bought four juicers–two for his house and two for the truck–two so that he'd always have a backup in case one broke down wherever he was. He also bought the longest extension cord he could find. He'd plug in the cord in restrooms at truck stops and juice on picnic tables. He said this was not easy because he'd often draw a crowd of folks who were very curious about what he was doing. They'd ask lots of questions and slow him down as he tried to explain what he was up to. But Dave never gave up. He just kept juicing and drinking his hearty green juice combinations on the road six days a week.

It paid off! Dave has lost well over 230 pounds. But that's not all. He has energy and vitality! He said he's noticed emotional changes as well as physical, such as feeling more loving toward people. Recently a friend told me she was standing near him at a raw foods lecture at Thrive Café–one of our local Seattle raw foods hangouts. "Dave was vibrating with energy," she said. "It was like he had electricity pumping through his body." (I think Dave was saturated with the vitality of raw plant life.)

I now say to people, "If Dave can juice on the road, living out of a truck most of the week, plugging in an extension cord in a restroom, and juicing on picnic tables, you can juice at home or at work." No more excuses!

Vegetable juice can also play an important role in stabilizing blood sugar, a vital factor in appetite control, because it's very low in sugar. Sugar and foods like refined flour products (such as bread, rolls, and pasta) that quickly turn into sugar in your body cause spikes and dips in blood sugar. Now that's something to get excited about. When your blood sugar gets low, you can get ravenously hungry and sometimes grouchy. The sugar percentage of vegetable juice is much lower than that of fruit juice and the calorie count is up to 50 percent less, yet the juice succeeds in satisfying a sweet tooth. Amazing! This makes vegetable juicing an absolute must for successful dieting. Experiment with carrot, lemon, and ginger or a combination of carrot, Jerusalem artichoke, lemon, and parsley juice when a carb-craving hits. The juice jolt will give those cravings a knockout!

Knock Out the Cravings!

We all know about cravings that kick up the appetite for things like chocolate chip cookies, ice cream, or tortilla chips. Experiencing strong food urges for sweets or salty snacks can feel almost as overwhelming as getting caught in a big ocean wave. The most frequently craved foods are usually high in sugar and unhealthy fat—the stuff that packs on the pounds big-time! We don't eat these foods for their nutritive value but usually for psychological reasons such as depression, disappointment, stress, or boredom. Or we may suffer from conditions like seasonal affective disorder (SAD) or PMS that cause us to want to clean out the fridge from time to time. Whatever it is that has you craving high-carb snacks, feeding your body super nutritious juices can make a huge difference in overcoming the hankering.

Vegetable juice helps curb your cravings because it's broken down into an easily absorbed form of nutrition that your body can quickly utilize. That means it doesn't have to go through the normal digestive process, which takes time. You can pack in a lot of food when you're really hungry before your brain kicks out the signal that there's enough nutrition to burn for energy. It's estimated that juice is at work in your system within about thirty minutes. Your body is supplied with supernutrients in short order. The signal goes to your brain that you're well fed and you no longer have the urge to eat.

Michelle Knocked Out Cravings With the Quickest Weight-Loss Plan Ever!

I've tried so many times to lose weight over the years. I've taken it off and put it back on more than once. The problem has been not being able to make a lifestyle change that I could live with and be consistent. I love to cook. I've found that I can get the same satisfaction out of choosing and juicing the right vegetables and fruit that I used to get from shopping and cooking. During the past three weeks,

I haven't experienced food cravings that I used to when I tried other diets. I look at this as a healthy eating change, not a diet. I've already gone down one dress size and can see a difference almost daily! This is by far the quickest weight loss that I've ever experienced. I wasn't even trying for that initially; I just wanted to feel better first. I got both at the same time.

—MICHELLE

When you satisfy your body with alkaline-rich, nutrient-dense juices and foods and your blood sugar stabilizes, your appetite for junk food, sweets, and high-carb fare begins to fade away. You may notice that your fatigue vanishes and energy zooms. You will feel more like getting up and going in the morning, working out, and getting things done. Like so many other juicing enthusiasts, you may also notice that your focus improves dramatically. That's because your brain is being well fed. When you eat nutrient-depleted food, your brain doesn't get as much of the raw materials it needs to make reactions happen. Things misfire, and you walk around looking for your car keys for ten minutes when they're in your pocket all the time. Now you can say good-bye to brain fog!

As you can see, there are a lot of benefits with the Turbo Diet. What other program can offer all of this?

Janice Lost 10 Pounds by Juicing and Cleansing

Let me first say a huge thank-you for all the work you do—for the books you've written and the many, many people you have helped, including myself. I feel very blessed to have been led to your juice book. I know I have embarked on a path that will be lifelong. I have been on every diet imaginable and every exercise program there is, and not one of them has had the impact on my life and my health like the information I got from you. I completed the liver cleanse and two weeks of the colon cleanse [from my book *Juicing, Fasting, and Detoxing for Life*]. It's amazing! I'm down 10 pounds. I'm loving every minute of the day—every mouthful of juice and food!

—JANICE

Boosting Your Metabolism

Metabolism begins the moment we're conceived and ends the moment we die. It is a constant and vital process for all life forms, not just human beings. If metabolism stops, death occurs.

In humans, metabolism begins with plants. A green plant takes in energy from sunlight. Photosynthesis then takes place as the plant uses this energy and chlorophyll to build nutrients from water and carbon dioxide.

When a person eats the plants or meat from animals that have eaten the plants, he or she absorbs this energy in the form of carbohydrates, along with other nutrients. Then the carbohydrates are broken down so that the energy can be distributed to the body's cells.

Glucagon is involved in the distribution of this energy. It's an important hormone involved in carbohydrate metabolism. Produced by the pancreas, it's released when blood glucose levels start to fall too low, causing the liver to convert stored glycogen into glucose and release it into the bloodstream. This raises blood glucose levels and ultimately prevents the development of low blood sugar. Glucagon also stimulates the release of insulin, so that newly available glucose in the bloodstream can be taken up and used by insulin-dependent cells.

The primary job of glucagon is to maintain stable blood sugar levels in the body by releasing stored body fat so it can be burned for energy. The pancreas, in response to protein, stimulates glucagon, which then stimulates the use of fat for energy. It shifts metabolism into a fat-burning mode and mobilizes the release of stored body fat from fat tissue directly into the bloodstream. This process allows muscles to burn fat instead of glucose for energy, converts dietary fats to ketones and sends them to the cells for energy, and releases fat from fat cells into the bloodstream for use. The result is effective weight management. When this system gets out of balance from consumption of too many simple and refined carbohydrates, we gain weight and find it hard to lose the extra pounds.

THE TURBO DIET IN A NUTSHELL

The Turbo Diet has payoffs with great dividends. I have personally witnessed people who have lost as much as a pound a day and without a lot of effort. There's no starvation, no deprivation.

Following are the basics of the program. (See the details of the complete program in chapter 7.) On the Turbo Diet, you will:

- Drink two glasses (10 to 12 ounces each) of fresh vegetable juice every day. If you don't have a juicer and can't afford to buy one right now, you can get premade juices at juice bars. If you don't have access to a juice bar, then you can purchase premade veggie juices from the cooler section of your grocery store. If those aren't available, then you can choose low-sodium V-8 juice. (Keep in mind that if the juice is bottled or canned, even if it's kept in the cooler section of a store, it has to be pasteurized. The heat used in pasteurization kills the vitamins, enzymes, and that mysterious life substance that you can only get in high measure in raw foods. You won't get the same effect from these juices as you do from fresh ones.) When you travel or it's not convenient to take juice along, you can get green powder, carrot powder, and beet powder to mix in water. (See Appendix A.)
- Eat a high-alkaline, low-glycemic diet. You will eat the largest portion of your foods from the alkaline-rich category consisting of vegetables, fruit, sprouts, nuts, seeds, healthy oils, and super greens. The rest of your diet will come from vegetarian or animal protein and a small amount of whole grains.
- Eat a large portion of your food raw—70 to 80 percent is your goal. Raw foods are loaded with enzymes and vitamins that are destroyed during cooking. Raw foods especially help you to lose weight.
- Eat plenty of vegetables on this diet, especially the brightly colored veggies that are highest in antioxidants. It is recommended that you consume at least two to three servings of veggies in addition to your vegetable juices.
- Eat small portions of lean protein—fish, chicken, turkey, lamb, beef, and eggs (if you don't choose to be vegan). Make these organic and free range for the healthiest choice.
- Drink eight to ten 8-ounce glasses of purified water each day. You could add some cranberry concentrate or pure unsweetened cranberry juice to the water to

improve flavor and help to get rid of stored-up water in your body. Cranberry is a natural diuretic, is helpful for kidney cleansing, and contains high levels of organic substances that are thought to have an emulsifying effect upon fat deposits.

- Drink a cup of green tea every day. Green tea is thermogenic, meaning that it helps to improve metabolism. If the caffeine in green tea (only about one-third that of coffee) does not agree with your system, then choose white tea (still has a little caffeine) or herbal tea. It's best to avoid coffee as much as possible since it's very acidic. It can also cause irritability and difficulty concentrating. Although coffee does rouse one a bit, later on it causes a collapse of energy, which can make you want to eat fattening food.

- Consume good fats such as avocado, extra-virgin olive oil, and virgin coconut oil. Coconut oil is a thermogenic; the liver likes to burn it. Contrary to popular opinion, it's a heart-healthy, slimming fat.

- Avoid starches, refined carbohydrates, sugar, sweets, alcohol, and sodas, including diet sodas.

- If you want the fast track, you can *juice fast* (some people call it *juice feast*) one day a week. That's where you drink just vegetable juices for a day. (See chapter 8 for the Turbo Diet Fast Menu Plan.) On these days you should drink around two quarts of vegetable juice. You could make one of the juice meals a raw energy soup (juice to which you add avocado; see page 144 for recipes) to help with energy and to stabilize blood sugar.

- You will also exercise three to four times per week.

Tips for Weight-Loss Success

- **Sleep enough; sleep well.** When we don't sleep enough or sleep well, our appetite-controlling hormones get out of whack and cause us to want to eat more, especially more carbohydrates. (If you need help with getting a good night's sleep, see chapter 5.)

- **Keep your colon moving.** Constipation can contribute to weight gain.

- **Keep well hydrated.** Some individuals end up in a state of chronic dehydration when they are trying to lose weight because they don't drink enough water; they are afraid of additional water weight. But they are actually hindering their bodies' ability to metabolize fat. A state of chronic dehydration will inevitably lead to weight gain. Being fully hydrated is a prerequisite to weight loss. To achieve successful weight loss, you must drink enough water so that your body is not in a state of chronic dehydration. When your body is in this state, you will not lose the excess fat very easily.

- **Keep a positive attitude.** Never tell yourself that you can't do something like lose weight. Remove all negative thoughts from your mind; speak and think only positive words to yourself and others. If you have a 5-pound reduction goal by the end of two weeks, see those 5 pounds gone. Think about this in terms of what you want to weigh by the end of two weeks. How great will you feel when you are 5 pounds lighter? Guard against self-defeat. Don't let it get you before you even get started.

If you reach a plateau at any time during your Turbo Diet or you want to accelerate your weight loss and healthy lifestyle plan, you can cleanse your body, starting with the colon cleanse program and then the seven-day Liver and Gallbladder Cleanse, which are outlined in detail in my books *Juicing, Fasting, and Detoxing for Life* and *The Juice Lady's Guide to Juicing for Health*. A congested liver and gallbladder could prevent you from losing weight. Also, you may find it impossible to shed pounds until you cleanse toxins from your body, especially the organs of elimination. For example, toxins trap water and fat cells in pockets we call cellulite. Detoxing your body is the key to ridding it of these lumpy fat deposits.

When you've lost most of the weight you want, you can slowly add in more healthy carbohydrates, including whole grains, potatoes, squash, and fruit. Typically, in this phase, you will lose about a pound per week. If you eat too many of these higher carb foods or you splurge for holidays, vacations, or special occasions and gain weight, you can quickly lose the extra pounds by cleansing your body with the One-Day Vegetable Juice Cleanse and strictly sticking with the Turbo Diet.

One day you will celebrate the achievement of your weight-loss goals. Then you will be able to eat more healthy carbohydrates, but you will be in the habit of choosing the right ones by this time. If you eat too much and put on a few pounds, you can get right back on track by going back to the Turbo Diet. If you trip up and binge during a stressful time, you can schedule a vegetable juice cleanse day and flush out the toxins. This is the design that can help you maintain your ideal weight for the rest of your life.

RESEARCH PROVES THE JUICE DIET WORKS!

Two university studies have shown that one to two glasses of vegetable juice a day promote four times the weight loss of non-juice drinkers on the same American Heart Association diet. Both studies were randomized controlled trials, each lasting twelve weeks.[1]

In the study conducted by University of California Davis among ninety healthy adults between the ages of forty and sixty-five, it was found that each person who drank at least two cups of vegetable juice a day met their weight-loss goal while only 7 percent of the non-juice drinkers met it. Participants who drank either one or two cups of vegetable juice per day lost an average of 4 pounds, while those who drank no vegetable juice lost only 1 pound. The researchers also found that people in the vegetable juice groups had significantly higher vitamin C and potassium intake and a significantly lower intake of carbohydrates. Participants with borderline high blood pressure who drank one or two servings of vegetable juice lowered their blood pressure significantly.[2]

The vegetable juice drinkers said they enjoyed the juice and felt like they were doing something good for themselves by drinking it. According to Carl Keen, PhD, professor of Nutrition and Internal Medicine at UC–Davis and coauthor of the study, "Enjoyment is so critical to developing good eating habits you can stick with for a long time.... Vegetable juice is something that people enjoy, plus it's convenient and portable, which makes it simple to drink every day."[3]

The Baylor College of Medicine study involved eighty-one adults who drank 8 to 16 ounces of vegetable juice daily as part of a calorie-controlled, heart-healthy diet. They showed an average of 4 pounds lost over a twelve-week study period compared with those who did not drink juice and lost only 1 pound. Of the participants in the study, almost three-quarters of whom were women, 83 percent had metabolic syndrome, which is a cluster of risk factors including excess body fat around the midsection, high blood pressure, high blood sugar, and elevated cholesterol.[4]

It is estimated that 47 million Americans have some combination of these risk factors, placing them at increased risk for diabetes and heart disease.[5] That's why the low-glycemic Turbo Diet works so well for weight loss and can be especially helpful for people with blood sugar challenges such as those with metabolic syndrome.

METABOLIC SYNDROME

Insulin is a powerful hormone, its primary job being to push glucose out of the blood and into cells where it's converted into energy. It plays a critical role in blood sugar balance, weight management, and other important health factors. When blood sugar goes up, the pancreas releases insulin to deal with the sugar, but it often overreacts by releasing too much insulin. Then your blood sugar drops down, often way down, and so you eat more carbohydrates to bring it up again. The pancreas releases more insulin—and on it goes.

Things like alcohol; pastries; candy; ice cream; pie; cake; refined flour products like bread, bagels, pizza, and pasta; and starches such as white potatoes and white rice rapidly break down to sugar and quickly enter the bloodstream where it causes insulin to spike. "It doesn't take much…to cause your blood sugar to skyrocket," says Ron Rosedale, MD. He notes that one saltine cracker can take blood sugar to over 100, and in many people it can cause it to go over 150.[6]

As insulin becomes overabundant, the normal target cells in the muscles and liver will no longer recognize it. When this happens on a continual basis, insulin floats in the bloodstream much of the time. When insulin becomes the dominant, active hormone, it triggers a hormone imbalance that sets the stage for weight gain, obesity, type 2 diabetes, and even cancer.

You Can't Maximize Fat Burning With Elevated Insulin Levels

Even if you exercise rigorously, elevated insulin levels will not maximize fat burning. Still worse, elevated insulin levels will stimulate your body to store fat. Remember, this response is primarily the result of eating too many carbohydrates and not enough protein, fat, and fiber, which are found in complex carbohydrates such as vegetables, legumes, and whole grains.

The key to correcting this imbalance begins with controlling insulin levels. Whether or not you have any of the symptoms of insulin resistance or metabolic syndrome, insulin control is vital for weight loss and maintenance. The low-glycemic diet with two glasses of vegetable juice per day is a good plan for you to control insulin response and maintain a lifetime of fitness.

Insulin carries glucose to the trillions of cells in your body. When you are insulin sensitive, your body will do a much better job of shuttling glucose (blood sugar) into your cells than when they are not sensitive to this hormone. The *open doors* of your cells allow this fuel to be used for energy. How easily glucose is shuttled into your cells defines how sensitive they are to insulin.

When your cells are not sensitive to insulin, insulin levels go up, and target cells will develop what is termed *insulin resistance*. When your cells are insulin resistant, your body must contend with extra "free-roaming" glucose that can't get into your cells. Some of this will be stored as fat and lead to weight gain. Without insulin sensitivity, you may struggle with your weight continually. Insulin resistance is thought to be one of the primary causes of overweight associated with metabolic syndrome.[7]

The Baylor College of Medicine study mentioned earlier involved a large percentage of participants with metabolic syndrome—a cluster of characteristics that include weight gain at the midsection, insulin resistance, low HDL, high blood pressure, and elevated triglycerides. If not corrected by following a low-glycemic diet, this syndrome usually evolves into diabetes. Most of the people with metabolic syndrome in the study lost weight when adding vegetable juice to their diet, four times the weight of others that did not drink juice. You can read more about this syndrome and how to correct it in chapter 5.

The Turbo Juice Diet Is Anti-Inflammatory

The standard Western diet produces inflammation. Inflammation produces insulin resistance. Insulin resistance produces weight gain. Weight gain produces inflammatory cytokines leading to more insulin resistance and more weight gain. It's a frustrating cycle. Insulin resistance starves the muscles, which react by sending signals to lower the metabolism to conserve energy reserves. Additionally, insulin resistance makes us hungry in an effort to feed our starving muscles.

Under these conditions, weight loss becomes almost impossible. We look overweight, but our muscles think we're starving. The sad fact is that many grossly overweight people are in fact starving. As a result of this starvation, we eat more and more food, but often we reach for the wrong foods—sugars, refined carbohydrates, simple starches, and unhealthy fats in response to brain signals calling for more nutrition. This impedes weight loss in spite of our best dieting efforts. As these conditions worsen, we may develop cardiovascular diseases, diabetes, and hypertension. The Turbo Diet halts the inflammatory response in its tracks, putting a stop to this cascade of unhealthy reactions, and turns the body around to a balanced biochemistry.

What Is the Low-Glycemic Diet?

The glycemic index (GI) has become a popular weight-loss tool based in part on the fact that high-glycemic foods raise blood sugar levels, cause the body to secrete excess insulin, and lead to the storage of fat. Originally developed to help diabetics manage blood sugar control, the glycemic index has become popular in the weight-loss market largely because it works so well. Researchers reported in the *Journal of the American Medical Association* that patients who lost weight with a low-glycemic diet kept the weight off longer than patients who lost the same amount of weight with a low-fat diet.[8]

The GI diet refers to a system of ranking carbohydrates according to how much a certain amount of each food raises a person's blood sugar level. It's determined by measuring how much a 50-gram serving of carbohydrate raises a person's blood sugar level compared with a control.

Virtually all carbohydrates are digested into glucose and cause a temporary rise in blood glucose levels, called the glycemic response. But some foods raise it more than others. This response is affected by many factors, including the quantity of food, the amount and type of carbohydrate, how it's cooked or eaten raw, and the degree of processing. Each food is assigned an index number from 1 to 100, with 100 as the reference score for pure glucose. Typically, foods are rated high (greater than 70), moderate (56–69), and low (less than 55).

Carolyn Lost 10 Pounds and Feels 100 Percent Better

Over the four-day Thanksgiving vacation I decided to try your low-glycemic diet. I am sixty-one years old and have survived cancer five times as well as chemotherapy, radiation, and nearly two dozen surgeries. I have serious radiation burns in my abdomen. It's also contributed to arthritis in my joints and legs. I wanted to lose some weight, but the most surprising thing is that about three days after I cleansed my system of the simple carbohydrates, the arthritis pain began to leave. I have not experienced arthritis pain for nearly four weeks now. I have lost 10 pounds and feel 100 percent better. I have researched many comments about your plan (which included coconut oil) and find nothing but fabulous reviews. This is a simple, easy, effective plan to follow.

—CAROLYN

Low-glycemic foods, especially raw vegetables, can help control blood sugar, appetite, and weight. Though helpful for everyone, they are especially helpful for people with type 2 diabetes, prediabetes, hypoglycemia, insulin resistance, and metabolic syndrome. Low-glycemic foods are absorbed more slowly, allowing a person to feel full longer and therefore less likely to overeat. Raw food experts such as Dr. John Douglas have found that raw carbohydrates such as the raw juices are better tolerated than cooked carbs. They don't elicit the addictive cravings that cooked foods cause. Douglas believes, as does the Finnish expert A. I. Virtanen, that the enzymes in raw food play an important role in the way they stimulate weight loss as they do in the treatment of obesity.[9]

On the Turbo Diet, you are encouraged to choose most of your carbohydrate foods from the low-glycemic index and a large percentage of those foods as raw. The foods on the recommended list on pages 128–137 are for the most part low glycemic and are nutrient-rich, not refined, and higher in fiber—like whole vegetables, fruit, and legumes (beans, lentils, split peas).

Not All Carbs Are Created Equal

Different carbohydrates take different pathways in the body after digestion. For example, some starchy foods are bound by an outer layer of very complex starches (fiber) like the legumes (beans, lentils, split peas), which increases the time it takes for them to be digested. So even though legumes are relatively high in carbohydrates, they have a lower glycemic response because of their complex encasing.

Carrots are another example of glycemic inconsistency; they're often referred to as a high-glycemic vegetable. If a person consumes 50 grams of carrots, which are required for the test, they've eaten about 5 cups of carrots. Not many of us would eat that many carrots, even when juicing them. And even in that high quantity, carrots are still in the low-glycemic category, just a little higher than many other vegetables.

There is also the antioxidant potential of foods to consider, meaning the amount of antioxidant nutrients a food contains, like beta-carotene and vitamin C that are abundant in many fruits and vegetables. In Chinese culture, carrots are often used as cooling medicine. Carrots, beets (both very rich in beta-carotene), and other brightly colored vegetables are especially important to include in our diet to prevent disease. These days many health professionals suggest we eliminate carrots and beets because of their glycemic rating, but the Turbo Diet does not exclude them because of their high nutrient and fiber content.

The Turbo Diet has eliminated foods that are higher on the glycemic index and foods that do not have fiber and turn to glucose rapidly. This diet also eliminates foods that aren't rich in nutrients. Also, fruit is limited in the beginning because of the higher sugar content and because many people suffer from yeast overgrowth (candidiasis), to which fruit sugar contributes.

Choosing low-glycemic foods that do not promote a rapid rise in insulin, and therefore do not promote fat storage, and foods that are rich in fiber and thus slow down the release of sugar into the bloodstream are the Turbo Diet's wise choices for weight loss.

In contrast, higher glycemic index foods will trigger a rise in blood sugar, followed by a drop in blood sugar and a cascade of hormonal changes, which tend to make you hungry again quickly. The higher glycemic index foods are metabolized more quickly than low-glycemic foods. The blood sugar spikes of high-glycemic foods cause particular problems for people with diabetes, prediabetes, hypoglycemia, and metabolic syndrome.

Quality, not quantity, of carbohydrates is the goal of the Turbo Diet. The aim is to feel full by enjoying plenty of smart carbs—like whole vegetables, limited amounts of whole grains, and legumes—along with lean protein, healthy fats, and a little fruit. You will completely avoid the high-glycemic foods, which tend to be made with sugar and/or white flour and are often highly processed.

THE GLYCEMIC INDEX REVIEW

The glycemic index was developed by David Jenkins in 1981 to measure the rise in blood glucose after consumption of a particular food. This index shows the rate at which carbohydrates break down to glucose in the bloodstream. Test subjects are given a specified amount (50 grams) of carbohydrates in a test food, and then their blood glucose is measured over a period of time to see how it is affected. The blood sugar response is compared to a standard food, usually white bread, and a rating is given to determine how blood sugar is affected.

Keep in mind that not all low-glycemic foods are healthy fare. Low-glycemic foods include candy bars and potato chips. These foods are not on the Turbo Diet because they are very nutrient depleted, contain sugar or turn to sugar easily, and lack fiber. You need to get the best nutrition for your choices. Likewise, there are moderate-scored foods such as beets and high-glycemic foods such as rutabagas and parsnips that are part of this plan because they are nutrient rich.

With this plan, there's no obsessing over the glycemic index either, just a basic understanding of the principles. Keep in mind that certain factors can change a score, such as the riper the fruit, the higher the glycemic index score. But always choose ripe fruits and vegetables over unripe; they are healthier by far. Adding good fat to foods can lower the GI score. And keep in mind that the GI response to any given food also varies widely from person to person. It can even vary within the same person from day to day.[10] That's why it's so important to be able to listen to your body and determine how the foods you are eating are affecting you.

Dmitriy Lost 40 Pounds

I lost 40 pounds mostly from around my waist over about a six-month period after I started juicing. I'm an athlete and used to working out a lot. But when I got a knee injury that prevented workouts, it became tougher to stay in shape. Then I started juicing every day. The weight just melted off without any effort. I went from a 38-inch waist to a 32-inch waist and from about 230 pounds to 190. I'm committed to juicing for the rest of my life.

—DMITRIY

WEIGHT LOSS ON A MISSION

Years ago when I was taking prerequisites for my masters of science program in whole foods nutrition at Bastyr University, I worked for a weight-loss center part-time as a nutrition counselor. I noticed that a number of people who entered the program looked healthy, meaning they had good skin color and tone and vibrancy—they were just overweight. Soon into the program, I noticed that though they were losing weight, they weren't looking healthier. I observed a loss of skin tone, skin color turning a grayish pallor, and a loss of energy and vitality. I was alarmed. Even as a student I knew that it was not just about dropping weight; it was about getting healthier. I quit the job, unable to promote something that I felt did harm.

Margo's Pain in Her Left Foot Is Gone!

Since I started juicing, my eyes are brighter and the pain in my left foot is gone! I could hardly walk before. I started juicing because I wanted to feel better and because I had lots of digestive problems. I had no idea that I would get rid of the pain in my left foot.

—MARGO

When you embark on a weight-loss program, it should be about getting healthier along with losing weight. Whether you want to lose 10, 20, 50, 100, or even more than 200 pounds like Dave the "Raw Foods" Trucker, it isn't just about getting the weight off any way you can. I know people who have lost weight through drastic means and ruined their health in the process.

Losing weight with vegetable juices and the Turbo Diet is one way to ensure that you choose a weight-loss regimen that doesn't sacrifice your health. That's why I'm excited about introducing you to the Turbo Diet. I know what it can do for you. So many people have praised this diet because of the increased health and energy they experienced. And if they can experience these great results, you can too. You're off to a great start and a lifetime of fitness!

Chapter 2

Juice Off the Pounds!

The TURBO DIET works! Now that you've read chapter 1, you know why it works. But just in case you're like me and need to hear things more than once, here's a review: It supplies an abundance of nutrients that satisfy the body's nutritional needs. That helps to squelch cravings—a huge plus for weight loss! It's energizing, so fatigue can become a thing of the past and you actually feel like working out. You build more muscle and burn more calories. It also detoxifies the body. Toxins can actually cause you to gain weight and make it very difficult to lose weight. This program is rich in foods that alkalinize the body. Drinking alkaline-rich juices encourages the body to burn fat cells with the acids they contain because there's plenty of buffer to neutralize the acids.

Now that you know in theory just how effective juicing is for weight loss, you will want to experience it firsthand. I'd like to help you get started on your turbo program with some guidelines for juicing and choosing a good juicer. I'll also give you answers to some frequently asked questions along with plenty of tips to make this a very easy plan to follow.

Karen Lost 20 Pounds!

I've lost about 20 pounds in five months. I started my new lifestyle with green smoothies, increased my vegetable intake, reduced my carbohydrates, added good oils, including virgin coconut oil, and ate lean meat and fish. Then I started juicing, which took me to a higher level of health. When I drink the juice, I feel better almost immediately. I notice when I don't drink it, my body starts to crave it.

My health has improved so much since I started the juice diet. My allergies decreased considerably when I started juicing. Once I changed my diet and started juicing, I had more of a desire to eat healthier. I now have more energy to get things done. I really like the energy the juice gives me. I make carrot and beet juice so I'll have energy to go exercise. This is a new thing for me to be able to exercise and not feel exhausted afterward. I love it.

I used to wake up in the morning really grumpy and more tired than when I went to bed. Now, on most days, I'm waking up happy and feeling better than ever. This is such a breakthrough for me. Even with the gloomy fall weather, I'm still really happy, and that makes my family a whole lot happier too.

At one point in my program, I just wasn't losing any more weight. Cherie suggested that I try a liver cleanse, which would help me get past the plateau. She also told me it would help me with my energy level. After about a week of being on her liver cleanse program, I could really feel a difference in the way I felt. I had more energy, and by the next week other symptoms cleared up, such as allergies to certain foods, dry lifeless hair, dull eyes, and spots on my skin. And I started losing weight again.

I wasn't sure at first how much Cherie's program would change my life, but now I am a true believer in juicing. Doing all this good stuff has given me a greater desire to want to eat healthier. It has also given me increased energy, decreased allergies, improved digestion, better health (not sick like I used to be), and I'm happier than ever before!

—Karen

*NOTE FROM AUTHOR: You can view Karen's before and after pictures at http://www.juiceladyinfo.com/weightLoss.shtml.

Juice Helps Control Your Appetite

Drinking a glass of vegetable juice before each meal can help curb your appetite. If you choose the ingredients with some care, you can get a double dividend of appetite control. The best vegetables to use when juicing for weight loss are *negative calorie foods*—those that require more calories to digest than they contain. Dark greens, broccoli, carrots, Jerusalem artichoke, fennel, and cabbage are among the best vegetables to use in juice recipes for weight loss. Also consider using asparagus, cucumber, and celery, which are natural diuretics that can alleviate water retention.

In addition, carrot juice and parsley juice can help to maintain blood sugar levels, which will help prevent hunger. Since carrot juice is sweet, it can also help to satisfy sugar cravings. Another vegetable to try for curing a sweet tooth is Jerusalem artichoke. However, although it reduces sugar cravings, Jerusalem artichoke is bland, so it's best combined with things like carrot, cucumber, and lemon juice to bring out its flavor.

Channah Lost 13 Pounds for Her Wedding

I lost a total of 13 pounds for my wedding and kept 8 pounds off by juicing. I attended one of Cherie's classes on juicing and cleansing and bought a juicer. Juicing has helped me keep the 8 pounds off. Beyond lost weight, I feel less sluggish and my complexion has improved. Overall I feel much more healthy. I really believe in juicing. Thanks, Cherie.

—Channah

*NOTE FROM AUTHOR: An exciting update is that Channah is now expecting a baby. She said she's more than gained back the weight she lost for her wedding, but she's looking forward to the Turbo Diet to get back in shape once her baby arrives.

Vegetable and Fruit Juices That Help Promote Weight Loss

Asparagus juice

Asparagus juice is a natural diuretic. It contains asparagine—a crystalline amino acid that boosts kidney performance, thereby improving waste removal from the body. You can juice the stems that you would normally throw away, which is good conservation of produce.

Beet juice

Beets are a natural diuretic that is also thought to help break up fatty deposits.

Cabbage juice

Cabbage is thought to aid in breakdown of fatty deposits, especially around the abdominal region.

Celery juice

Celery juice is a diuretic and has calming properties. Celery is also good source of natural sodium.

Cranberry juice

Cranberries are a diuretic. Juice up cranberries with lemon and a low-sugar green apple; it tastes like lemonade and makes a delicious weight-loss treat.

Cucumber juice

Cucumbers help increase urination and aid in flushing out toxins. Cucumbers are rich in sulfur and silicon, which stimulate the kidneys to better remove uric acid. The silicon is also great for hair and nails and helps to prevent hair loss and nail splitting.

Tomato juice

Tomatoes contain citric acid and malic acid, which enhance the body's metabolism, promoting more efficient calorie burning.

Robin Lost 9 Pounds in One Week

Well, to my surprise, this Saturday morning I weighed myself, and I was 9 pounds LESS than I was on Sunday night! WOO HOO! I know I have a ways to go, but to have gone that far in just a week seemed absolutely unfathomable! I did an exercise program at a club for over a year but did not lose a single pound. I know that exercise is important. But my biggest problem was not being dealt with–the food. I did not want to deal with it; it was too hard. This week I did not stress exercise. I did walk around the church field before Bible study on Wednesday night, but that was all. I knew I would lose some weight this week. I was determined! But to lose 9 pounds just amazes me. And to top that off, the pain in my foot is gone. I had plantars fasciitis, which made it painful to walk and very difficult to exercise. It's just amazing that this pain is gone. I can now go for walks and keep moving.

—ROBIN

FRESH JUICE OFFERS A CORNUCOPIA OF NUTRIENTS

Every time you pour a glass of juice, picture a big vitamin-mineral cocktail with a cornucopia of the nutrients that promote weight loss and vitality. In addition to water and easily absorbed protein and carbohydrates, known as macronutrients (the ones we need in larger quantity), juice also provides some essential fatty acids and loads of vitamins, minerals, enzymes, and phytonutrients. And researchers are continuing to explore how the nutrients found in juice help the body heal and shed unwanted pounds.

The next time you make a glass of fresh juice, this is what you will be drinking:

Protein

Did you ever consider juice to be a source of protein? Surprisingly, it does offer more than you might think. We use protein to form muscles, ligaments, tendons, hair, nails, and skin. Protein is necessary to create enzymes, which direct chemical reactions, and hormones, which pilot bodily functions. Fruits and vegetables contain lower quantities of protein than animal foods, such as muscle meats and dairy products, and they are incomplete proteins. Therefore, they are thought of as poor protein sources. But juices are concentrated forms of vegetables and so provide easily absorbed amino acids, the building blocks that make up protein. For example, 16 ounces of carrot juice (2–3 pounds of carrots) provides about 5 grams of protein (the equivalent of about one chicken wing or a small egg). In addition to juicing plenty of dark leafy greens and root vegetables like carrots and beets, you will want to eat other protein sources, such as sprouts, legumes (beans, lentils, and split peas), nuts, seeds, and whole grains. If you're not vegan, you can add eggs and free-range, grass-fed muscle meats such as chicken, turkey, lamb, and beef, along with wild-caught fish.

Carbohydrates

Vegetable juice contains healthy carbohydrates. Carbs provide fuel for the body, which it uses for movement, heat production, and chemical reactions. The chemical bonds of carbohydrates lock in the energy a plant takes up from the sun (photosynthesis), and this energy is released when the body burns plant food as fuel. There are three categories of carbs: simple (sugars), complex (starches and fiber), and fiber. Choose more complex carbohydrates in your diet over simple carbs. There are more simple sugars in fruit juice than vegetable juice, which is why you should juice vegetables and eat the fruit whole, except for lemon, lime, and low-sugar apple, which you can use to flavor vegetable juice recipes. Both insoluble fiber and soluble fiber are found in whole fruits and vegetables; both types are needed for good health. But who said juice doesn't have fiber? Juice has the soluble form, which is excellent for the digestive tract. Soluble fiber also helps to lower blood cholesterol levels, stabilize blood sugar, and improve good bowel bacteria.

Essential fatty acids

There is very little fat in fruit and vegetable juices, but the fats juice does contain are essential to your health. The fatty acids linoleic and alpha-linolenic (an omega-3 fat) are found in fresh vegetable juice. They support the cardiovascular, reproductive, immune, and nervous systems. They are also required for energy production.

Vitamins

Fresh juice is replete with vitamins. Vitamins take part, along with minerals and enzymes, in chemical reactions throughout the body. For example, vitamin C is helpful for weight loss in that it's involved in the proper conversion of glucose to energy in the cells. Dark leafy greens and citrus are rich in vitamin C. Vitamin B_5 is involved in the utilization of fat. It also plays an important role in energy production and assists adrenal function. It's found in dark leafy greens. Fresh juice is an excellent source of water-soluble vitamins like C, many of the B vitamins, some fat-soluble vitamins such as the carotenes (also known as provitamin A, which are converted to vitamin A as needed), and vitamins E and K. They also come packaged with cofactors that enhance their effectiveness to work together, such as vitamin C with bioflavonoids. The bioflavonoids make vitamin C more effective.

Minerals

Fresh juice is loaded with minerals. There are seven major minerals that the body needs; it also utilizes over eighty minerals to maintain good health. Minerals, along with vitamins, are components of enzymes. They make up bone, teeth, and blood tissue, and they help maintain normal cellular function. Some minerals are important for weight loss. For example, calcium works with certain amino acids to regulate fat metabolism and prevent fat storage. Magnesium increases calcium absorption. And chromium works with insulin to help the body use blood sugar.

Minerals occur in inorganic forms in the soil, and plants incorporate them into their tissues. As a part of this process, the inorganic minerals are converted to organic minerals through a process called photosynthesis, which produces minerals in an absorbable form. This makes plant food an excellent dietary source of minerals. Juicing is believed to provide even better mineral absorption than whole vegetables because the process of juicing liberates minerals into a highly absorbable, easily digested state.

Enzymes

Fresh juice is chock-full of enzymes, which are biological catalysts that speed up specific chemical reactions in a cell. They work, often with vitamins and minerals, to speed up reactions necessary for vital functions in the body. Without enzymes, we would not have life in our cells. Enzymes are prevalent in raw foods and juice, but heat, such as cooking and pasteurization, destroys them. All juices that are bottled, even if kept in refrigerators, have to be pasteurized. Temperature for pasteurization is required to be far above the limit of what would preserve the enzymes and vitamins.

When you eat and drink enzyme-rich juice and foods, these little catalysts help break down food in the digestive tract, thereby sparing digestive organs such as the pancreas, liver, and gallbladder—the body's enzyme-producers—from overwork. This sparing action is known as the "law of adaptive secretion of digestive enzymes." According to this law, when the food you eat is processed by enzymes present in the food you ingest, the body will secrete less of its own enzymes. This allows the body's energy to be shifted from digestion to other functions such as repair and rejuvenation.

Enzymes are vitally important for weight loss. For example, the enzyme lipase is a fat-splitting enzyme that is found abundantly in raw, live foods. However, few of us eat enough raw foods to get enough lipase to burn even a normal amount of fat, not to mention any excess. Lipase helps the body in digestion, fat distribution, and fat burning for energy. Lipase breaks down fat throughout the body. Without lipase, fat accumulates, and we can see it collecting on our hips, thighs, buttocks, and stomach. Protease is an enzyme that helps break down proteins and eliminate toxins. Eliminating toxins is essential when we're burning fat. The body stores excess toxins in fat cells. As we begin to burn fat, toxins are released into our system. This can sometimes cause water retention and bloating. It's important to have plenty of protease when losing weight.

Phytochemicals

Plants contain substances that protect them from disease, injury, and pollution. These substances are known as phytochemicals—*phyto* means plant, and *chemical* in this context means nutrient. These health-protecting compounds are found in fruits, vegetables, and other plants. Phytochemicals (sometimes called phytonutrients) include beta-carotene, lycopene, and resveratrol. They give plants their color, odor, and flavor. Unlike vitamins and enzymes, they are heat stable and can withstand cooking. Certain phytochemicals, such as indole-3-carbinol, target release and metabolism of stored fat. Also, researchers have found that people who eat the most fruits and vegetables have the lowest incidence of cancer and other diseases.[1] Drinking vegetable juices gives you these vital substances in a highly absorbable, concentrated form.

Light energy

There's one more substance, more difficult to measure than the others, that's present in raw foods. Light energy is found in the living cells of raw foods such as fruits and vegetables. They have been shown to emit coherent light rays when uniquely photographed (in Kirlian photography). This light energy is believed to have many benefits when consumed; one in particular is thought to aid cellular communication. It's also believed to contribute to our energy, vitality, and a feeling of vibrancy and well-being.

Vitalism is a word that means vital spark or energy. It was a hypothesis that was debated in the seventeenth to nineteenth centuries. Vitalism has a long history in medical philosophies. Most traditional healing practices put forward that disease was the result of some imbalance in the vital energies. As medicine became more mechanistic in the twentieth century, the concept of vitalism, or vital spark, fell out of vogue. However, it is the vital spark of life that is in raw vegetables and fruit that gives life to the body. This may be one reason that people report a significant increase in energy when they start drinking fresh juice.

FREQUENTLY ASKED QUESTIONS ABOUT JUICING

Now that you know why juice is so effective for weight loss and so good for your health, you may have some questions about juicing. Following are some of the most commonly asked questions:

Why juice? Why not just eat the fruits and vegetables?

Although I'd never tell anyone not to eat their vegetables and fruit, there are at least three reasons why juicing is important and should also be included in your diet. First, you can juice (and drink) far more produce than you would probably eat in a day. It takes a long time to chew raw veggies. Chewing is a very good thing. I highly encourage it. However, there's only so much time you have for chewing up raw foods. One day I timed how long it would take for me to eat five medium-size carrots. (That's what I often juice along with cucumber, lemon, ginger-root, beet, kale, and celery.) It was about fifty minutes of chewing. Not only do I not have that kind of time every day, but also my jaw was so tired afterward that I could hardly move it.

Secondly, we can juice parts of the plant we would not normally eat, such as stems, leaves, peels, and seeds. I juice things I know I would rarely or never eat such as beet stems and leaves, celery leaves, the white pithy part of the lemon and lime with the seeds, asparagus stems, and kale leaves with the rib.

Thirdly, it's estimated that juice is at work in the system in about twenty to thirty minutes after drinking it. And for ailments, juice is therapy for this very reason. When the body has to work hard to break down veggies, for example, it can spend a lot of energy on the digestive process. Juicing does the work for you. So when you drink a glass of fresh juice, all those life-giving nutrients can go to work right away to energize, heal, and repair your body.

What about the fiber that's lost in juicing?

It's true that we need to eat whole vegetables, fruit, sprouts, legumes, and whole grains for fiber. We drink juice for the extra nutrients; it's better than any vitamin pill. And for weight loss, we drink vegetable juices for appetite control. I also recommend juice as therapy in my book *The Juice Lady's Guide to Juicing for Health.* Don't worry about the fiber that is lost when you juice; you still get soluble fiber in the juice. And think about all the extra nutrition you're getting. Fresh juice is one of the best vitamin/mineral cocktails you could drink. You may not need as many nutritional supplements when you juice, so that could save you a lot of money in the long run. Drink your juice as a smart addition to your high-fiber diet that you will get from raw foods, legumes, sprouts, fruits, and vegetable dishes.

Do many of the nutrients remain with the fiber?

In the past, some health-minded groups have thought that a significant amount of nutrients stayed in the fiber after juicing, but that theory has been disproved. The U.S. Department of Agriculture (USDA) analyzed twelve fruits and found that 90 percent of the antioxidant nutrients they measured was in the juice rather than the fiber.[2] That is why juice makes such a great supplement in the diet.

Is fresh juice better than commercially processed juice?

Fresh juice is "live food" with a full complement of vitamins, minerals, phytochemicals, and enzymes, along with light energy. In contrast, commercially processed canned, bottled, frozen, or packaged juices have been pasteurized, which means the juice has been heated and many of the vitamins and enzymes have been killed or removed. And the light energy is virtually gone. Look at a Kirlian photograph of a cooked vegetable or a pasteurized glass of juice, and you will see very little "light" emanating from them. This means the juice will have longer shelf life, but it won't give your body the kind of life you will get from raw juice. Making your own juice also allows you to choose organic produce and to use a wider variety of vegetables and fruit you might not otherwise eat like kale, beets with leaves and stems, lemon with the white part, and chunks of gingerroot. Some of my recipes include Jerusalem artichokes, jicama, green cabbage, beet with stem and leaves, celery leaves, kale, and parsley. These sweet, crisp tubers and healthy greens are not found in most processed juices.

How long can you store fresh juice?

The sooner you drink juice after you make it, the more nutrients you will get. However, you can store juice and not lose too many nutrients by keeping it cold, such as in an insulated container or in a covered jar in the refrigerator. If you fill the container up to the top and get rid of as much air as possible, you will have less oxidation.

On a personal note: When I had chronic fatigue syndrome, I would juice in the afternoons, when I had the most energy, and store the juice covered in the refrigerator and drink it for the next twenty-four hours until I juiced my next batch of juice. I got well doing that. You can read more about my journey to health in *The Juice Lady's Guide to Juicing for Health*.

How much produce is needed to make a glass of juice?

People often ask me if it takes a "bushel basket" of produce to make a glass of juice. Actually, if you're using a good juicer, it takes a surprisingly small amount of produce. For example, all of the following items, each weighing roughly a pound, yield about one 8-ounce glass of juice: one medium apple, one-half cucumber, and one-half lemon (combined); five to seven carrots; or one large cucumber. The following each yield about 4 ounces of juice: three large (13-inch) stalks of celery or one orange. The key is to get a good juicer that yields a dry pulp. I've used juicers that ejected very wet pulp. When I ran the pulp through the juicer again, I got a lot of juice and the pulp was still wet. If the rpm is too high or the juicer is not efficient in other ways, you will waste a lot of produce.

Will juicing cost a lot of money?

People often wonder just how expensive is it to make a glass of juice. You can figure the cost of an 8-ounce glass is often less than a latte. With three or four carrots, half a lemon, a chunk of gingerroot, two stalks of celery, and half a cucumber, you will probably spend two and a half dollars to three and a half dollars, depending on the season, the area of the country, and the store where you shop. There are also hidden savings. You may not need as many vitamin supplements. What's that worth? And you will probably need far less over-the-counter medications like painkillers; sleeping aids; antacids; and cold, cough, and flu medications. That's a whopping savings! And then there's time not lost from work. What happens when you run out of sick days? Or if you're self-employed, you've missed out on income each day you're sick. With the immune-building, disease-fighting properties of fresh juice, you should stay well all year long.

How to Choose the Right Juicer

Choosing a juicer that is right for you can make the difference between juicing daily and never juicing again, so it's important to get one that works for your lifestyle.

People often ask me if they can use their blender as a juicer. You can't use a blender to make juice. A juicer separates the liquid from the pulp (insoluble fiber). A blender liquefies everything that is placed in it; it doesn't separate the insoluble fiber from the juice. If you think it might be a good idea to have carrot, beet, parsley, or celery pulp in your juice for added fiber, I can tell you from experience that it tastes like juicy sawdust. For the most flavorful juice, which is juice you'll enjoy and drink every day, you need a juicer. Look for the following features:

- *Has adequate horsepower (hp).* I recommend a juicer with 0.3 to 0.5 hp. Weak-motored machines with low horsepower ratings must run at an extremely high rpm (revolutions per minute). A machine's rpm does not accurately reflect its ability to perform effectively because rpm is calculated when the juicer is running idle, not while it is juicing. When you feed produce into a low-power machine, the rpm will be reduced dramatically, and sometimes the juicer will come to a full stop. I have "killed" some machines on the first carrot I juiced.

- *Is efficient at extracting juice.* I have used a number of juicers that wasted a lot of produce because there was a lot of juice left in the pulp. You should not be able to squeeze juice out of the pulp. Some machines have too high an rpm, and the pulp comes out very saturated with juice. I've had people tell me they were spending a lot of money on produce, which should not be the case. It often turned out that they were wasting a lot of produce because of an inefficient juicer.

- *Sustains blade speed during juicing.* Look for a machine that has electronic circuitry that sustains blade speed during juicing.

- *Is able to juice all types of produce.* Make sure the machine can juice tough, hard produce, such as carrots and beets, as well as delicate greens, such as parsley, lettuce, and herbs. Make sure it doesn't need a special citrus attachment. For wheatgrass juice, you will need a wheatgrass juicer or a juicer that presses the juice such as a single or double auger machine, also known as a masticating juicer. Be aware that the machines that juice wheatgrass along with other vegetables and fruit take more time to use. Most of them have a small opening, which means you will have to chop your produce in small pieces. (You don't have to do this with a wide-mouth juicer.) Some are more time consuming to clean as well.

- *Has a large feed tube, known as a wide-mouth juicer.* If you don't have a lot of time to devote to juicing, make sure you get a wide-mouth machine. Cutting your produce into small pieces before juicing does take extra time.

- *Ejects pulp.* Choose a juicer that ejects pulp into a receptacle. This design is far better than one in which all the pulp stays inside the machine and has to be scooped out frequently. Juicers that keep the pulp in the center basket rather than ejecting it cannot juice continuously. You will need to stop the machine often to wash it out. Plus, you can line the pulp catcher with a free plastic baggie from the grocery store produce section and you won't have to wash the receptacle each time. When you're finished juicing, you can either toss the pulp or use it in cooking or composting, but you won't need to wash this part of the juicer.

- *Has only a few parts to clean.* Look for a juicer with only a few parts to clean. The more parts a juicer has and the more complicated the parts are to wash, the longer it will take to clean up and the more time it will take to put it back together. That makes it less likely you will use your machine daily. Also, make sure the parts are dishwasher safe. I just rinse the juicer I use and let it air dry.

For recommendations on juicers, see Appendix A.

How to Get the Most From Juicing

Juicing is a very simple process. Simple as the procedure is, though, it helps to keep a few guidelines in mind to get the best results.

- *Wash all produce before juicing.* Fruit and vegetable washes are available at many grocery and health food stores. Cut away all moldy, bruised, or damaged areas of the produce.

- *Always peel oranges, tangerines, tangelos, and grapefruit* before juicing because the skins of these citrus
  fruit contain volatile oils that can cause digestive
  problems like a stomachache. Lemon and lime peels
  can be juiced, if organic, but they do add a distinct
  flavor that is not one of my favorites for most recipes.
  I usually peel them. Leave as much of the white pithy
  part on the citrus fruit as possible, since it contains the
  most vitamin C and bioflavonoids. Bioflavonoids work
  with vitamin C; they need each other to create the best
  uptake for your immune cells. Always peel mangoes
  and papayas, since their skins contain an irritant that is
  harmful when eaten in quantity.

  Also, I recommend that you peel all produce that is
  not labeled organic, even though the largest concentration of nutrients is in and next to the skin. For
  example, nonorganic cucumbers are often waxed,
  trapping the pesticides. You don't want the wax or the
  pesticides in your juice. The peels and skins of sprayed
  fruits and vegetables contain the largest concentration
  of pesticides.
- *Remove pits, stones, and hard seeds* from such fruits as
  peaches, plums, apricots, cherries, and mangoes. Softer
  seeds from cucumbers, oranges, lemons, limes, water-
  melons, cantaloupes, grapes, and apples can be juiced
  without a problem. Because of their chemical composition, large quantities of apple seeds should not be juiced
  for young children under the age of two, but they should
  not cause problems for older children and adults.
- *You can juice the stems and leaves* of most produce
  such as beet stems and leaves, strawberry caps, celery
  leaves, and small grape stems; stems offer nutrients too.
  Discard larger grape stems, as they can dull the juicer
  blade. Also remove carrot and rhubarb greens because
  they contain toxic substances. Cut off the ends of
  carrots since this is the part that molds first.
- *Cut fruits and vegetables* into sections or chunks that
  will fit your juicer's feed tube. You will learn from
  experience what can be added whole or what size works

best for your machine. If you have a large feed tube,
you won't have to cut up a lot of produce.

- *Some fruits and vegetables don't juice well.* Most
  produce contains a lot of water, which is ideal for
  juicing. Vegetables and fruits that contain less water,
  such as bananas, mangoes, papayas, and avocados,
  will not juice well. They can be used in smoothies and
  cold soups by first juicing other produce, then pouring
  the juice into a blender, and adding the avocado, for
  example, to make a raw soup.
- *Drink your juice as soon as you can after it's made.* If
  you can't drink the juice right away, store it in an insulated container such as a stainless steel water bottle,
  thermos, or another airtight, opaque container, and in
  the refrigerator if possible, for up to twenty-four hours.
  Light, heat, and air will destroy nutrients quickly. Be
  aware that the longer juice sits before you drink it,
  the more nutrients are lost. If juice turns brown, it
  has oxidized and lost a large amount of its nutritional
  value. After twenty-four hours, it may become spoiled.
  Melon and cabbage juices do not store well; drink them
  soon after they've been juiced.

Choose Organic Produce

The popularity of organic foods has increased dramatically in recent
years, and it continues to grow. Sales of organic foods reach into the
billions of dollars each year and continue to increase annually. It appears
that an ever-growing number of people want to avoid the billion pounds
or more of pesticides and herbicides sprayed onto or added to our crops
yearly. That's for good reason! It's estimated that a small percentage of
pesticides actually fights insects and weeds, while the rest is absorbed
into the plants and diffused into our air, soil, and water.

There are concerns that pesticides used to control pests on food
crops are dangerous to people who consume those foods. These
concerns are one reason for the organic food movement. Many food
crops, including fruits and vegetables, contain pesticide residues after
being washed or peeled. Chemicals that are no longer used but that are
resistant to breakdown for long periods may remain in soil and water
and thus in food.[3] These pesticide residues pose long-term health risks,

such as cancer and birth defects.[4] A study conducted by the Harvard School of Public Health in Boston has discovered a 70 percent increase in the risk of developing Parkinson's disease for people exposed to even low levels of pesticides.[5] There are immediate health risks for people who work with pesticides, such as acute intoxication, vomiting, diarrhea, blurred vision, tremors, convulsions, and nerve damage.

If pesticides and herbicides do not (as we're told), pose a health risk, then why is there is a greater incidence of cancer among farmers? There have been many studies of farmers intended to determine health effects of occupational pesticide exposure. Associations between non-Hodgkin's lymphoma, leukemia, prostate cancer, multiple myeloma, and soft tissues sarcoma have been reported.[6]

I'm often asked if organic produce is more nutritious than conventionally grown produce. Studies have shown that it is. According to results from a $25 million study into organic food, the largest of its kind to date, organic produce completely outshines conventional produce in nutritional content. A four-year, European Union–funded study found that organic fruits and vegetables contain up to 40 percent more antioxidants. They have higher levels of beneficial minerals like iron and zinc. Milk from organic herds contained up to 90 percent more antioxidants. The researchers obtained their results after growing fruits and vegetables, and raising cattle, on adjacent organic and nonorganic sites attached to Newcastle University. According to Professor Carlo Leifert, coordinator of the project, eating organic foods can even help to increase the nutrient intake of people who don't eat the recommended number of servings of fruits and vegetables a day.[7]

Additionally, a 2001 study completed as part of a doctoral dissertation at Johns Hopkins University looked at forty-one different studies involving field trials, greenhouse pot experiments, market basket surveys, and surveys of farmers. The most studied nutrients across those surveys included calcium, copper, iron, magnesium, manganese, phosphorus, potassium, sodium, zinc, beta-carotene, and vitamin C. According to the study, there was significantly more vitamin C (27 percent), iron (21 percent), magnesium (29 percent), and phosphorus (13 percent) in the organic produce than in the conventionally grown vegetables. There were also 15 percent fewer nitrates in the organic vegetables. The vegetables that had the biggest increases in nutrients between organic and conventional production were lettuce, spinach, carrots, potatoes, and cabbage.[8] Couple that with fewer chemical residues, and you can see that buying organically grown food is well worth the effort and the additional cost.

When choosing organically grown foods, look for labels that are marked *certified organic*. This means the produce has been cultivated according to strict uniform standards that are verified by independent state or private organizations. Certification includes inspection of farms and processing facilities, detailed record keeping, and pesticide testing of soil and water to ensure that growers and handlers are meeting government standards. You may occasionally see a label that says *transitional organic*. This means that the produce was grown on a farm that recently converted or is in the process of converting from chemical sprays and fertilizer to organic farming.

You may not be able to afford to purchase everything organic. When that's the case, choose wisely. According to the Environmental Working Group, commercially farmed fruits and vegetables vary in their levels of pesticide residue. Some vegetables (like broccoli, asparagus, and onions) as well as foods with thicker peels (such as avocados, bananas, and oranges) have relatively low levels of pesticides compared to other fruits and vegetables.[9] Be aware that some vegetables and fruits contain large amounts of pesticide. Each year the Environmental Working Group releases their list of the "Dirty Dozen" fruits and vegetables and rates fruits and vegetables from worst to best. You can check it out online at www.ewg.org.

When organic vegetables or fruit that you want are not available, ask your grocer to get them. You can also look for small-operation farmers in your area and check out farmers markets in season. Many small farms can't afford to use as many chemicals in farming as large commercial farms use. Another option is to order organic produce by mail.

Two Foods That Are Organic "Must-Buys"

1. *Potatoes* are an essential part of the American diet. One survey found they account for 30 percent of our overall vegetable consumption. A simple switch to organic potatoes has the potential to have a big impact because commercially farmed potatoes are some of the most pesticide-contaminated vegetables. A 2006 USDA test found 81 percent of potatoes tested still contained pesticides after being washed and peeled, and the potato has one of the highest pesticide contents of 43 fruits and vegetables tested, according to the Environmental Working Group.[10]

2. *Apples:* Apples are the second most commonly eaten

fresh fruit, after bananas, and they are the second most popular fruit juice, after oranges. But apples are also one of the most pesticide-contaminated fruits. The good news is that organic apples are easy to find, not overly expensive, and readily available in most grocery stores.

AVOID THE "DIRTY DOZEN"

If you can't afford to purchase all organic produce, you could still avoid the worst pesticide-sprayed offenders by buying only organically grown produce for the foods on the top-contaminated list. The nonprofit research organization Environmental Working Group reports periodically on health risks posed by pesticides in produce. The group says you can cut your pesticide exposure by almost 90 percent simply by avoiding the twelve conventionally grown fruits and vegetables that have been found to be the most contaminated. It has been found that eating the twelve most contaminated fruits and vegetables will expose a person to about fourteen pesticides per day, on average. Eating the twelve least contaminated will expose a person to less than two pesticides per day.[11] The list changes each year. To get the current ratings, got to www.ewg.org. As of this book's printing, here are the Environmental Working Group's "Dirty Dozen" and "Clean 15."[12]

ENVIRONMENTAL WORKING GROUP'S "DIRTY DOZEN"

Rank	Fruit or Veggie	Score The ratings below are from the worst contaminated fruits and vegetables to the lesser contaminated. On this list, peaches are the worst at 100, followed by other fruits and vegetables in descending order. It is recommended that you buy these foods only as organically grown.
1 (worst)	Peach	100 (highest pesticide load)
2	Apple	93
3	Sweet bell pepper	83
4	Celery	82
5	Nectarine	81
6	Strawberries	80
7	Cherries	73
8	Kale	69
9	Lettuce	67
10	Grapes (imported)	66
11	Carrot	63
12	Pear	63

ENVIRONMENTAL WORKING GROUP'S "CLEAN 15"

Rank	Fruit or Veggie	Score *The following items are rated beginning with the cleanest. They are all in the low category, meaning that choosing organic isn't as imperative with these foods.*
1	Onion	1 (lowest pesticide load)
2	Avocado	1 (lowest pesticide load)
3	Sweet corn (frozen)	2
4	Pineapple	7
5	Mango	9
6	Asparagus	10
7	Sweet peas (frozen)	10
8	Kiwi	13
9	Cabbage	17
10	Eggplant	20 .
11	Papaya	20
12	Watermelon	26
13	Broccoli	28
14	Tomato	29
15	Sweet potato	29

SHOULD WE EAT IRRADIATED FOOD?

Food irradiation exposes food to ionizing radiation in order to destroy microorganisms, bacteria, viruses, or insects that might be present in the food. Stay away from irradiated fruits and vegetables as much as possible. Some food producers use gamma-ray radiation to kill pests, bacteria, and germs in stored food and to increase the food's shelf life. Dr. George Tritsch of Roswell Park Memorial Institute, New York State Department of Health, says he is opposed to consuming irradiated food "because of the abundant and convincing evidence in scientific literature that the condensation products of the free radicals formed during irradiation produce statistically significant increases in carcinogenesis, mutagenesis, and cardiovascular disease in animals and man." There is also reported destruction of vitamins and other nutrients.[13] This practice destroys phytochemicals and enzymes, and it also generates harmful by-products such as free radicals, which are toxic and can damage cells, and harmful chemicals known as *radiolytic products*, including thalidomide.[14] Irradiation of fruits and vegetables may pose an even greater problem than irradiation of other foods due to the large quantities of water found in produce, which allows for greater free-radical production.

The answer to food-borne illnesses is not irradiation but stopping the overuse of pesticides, transforming overcrowded factory-farm animal lots to humane farms, and ensuring more sanitary conditions in food-processing plants.

AVOID GM FOODS

Whenever possible, you should avoid genetically modified foods, also know as GMs or GMOs. GMOs (genetically modified organisms) are the result of laboratory techniques by which researchers change plant and farm animal genes to create products with scientifically manufactured proteins or other substances that the human body has no prior experience digesting. Genetically modified plants, for example, may contain non-plant genetic material that may cause the plant to make never-before-encountered chemicals, which the body is unable to deal with. The altering of plant genes has been done to make plants more resistant to pests, disease, or pesticides; to have a longer shelf life; or to modify ripening.

A recent study revealed that experiments carried out by Monsanto researchers on three strains of GM maize (corn) showed signs of liver and kidney damage in test animals. Two of the varieties of maize were genetically modified to synthesize toxins used as insecticides, while the third was genetically modified to be resistant to the herbicide Roundup.[15] All three strains of the genetically modified corn are grown and approved for human consumption in America. According to various reports, Monsanto released the raw data only after a legal challenge from Greenpeace and other governmental bodies and groups against genetically modified foods.[16]

In the study, there were unusual concentrations of hormones in the blood and urine of rats fed the maize (each strain) for three months, compared to rats given a non-GM diet. Female rats were found to have higher levels of blood sugar and triglycerides. This finding is particularly significant regarding weight loss because it is known that higher blood sugar levels and triglycerides contribute to insulin resistance and metabolic syndrome, which was discussed in chapter 1. The authors of the study concluded, "Effects were mostly associated with the kidney and liver, the dietary detoxifying organs, although different between the three GMOs. Other effects were also noticed in the heart, adrenal glands, [and] spleen."[17]

Many genetically modified foods are on grocery store shelves everywhere without protective labeling. We may not know we are buying them. And unsuspecting consumers who may have an allergic reaction to something such as a peanut or Brazil nut may buy a product with a nut gene that could cause a life-threatening reaction.

We can avoid GMO foods by becoming aware of which foods are most prone to genetic engineering and what products are made from them. Some estimates say that as many as thirty thousand different products on grocery store shelves are "modified." That's largely because many processed foods contain some form of soy. About 90 percent of North America's soy crop is genetically engineered.[18] According to the FDA, more than fifty plant varieties have been examined and approved for human consumption[19]—for example, tomatoes and cantaloupes, modified ripening characteristics; soybeans and sugar beets, resistant to herbicides; corn and cotton plants, increased resistance to insect pests. While all fifty products may not be available in your local supermarket, the prevalence of genetically modified foods in the United States is more widespread than you may think. Deborah Whitman of Cambridge Scientific Abstracts states, "Highly processed foods, such as vegetable oils or breakfast cereals, most likely contain a small percentage of genetically modified ingredients because the raw ingredients have been pooled into one processing stream from many different sources."[20]

Worldwide, soybeans and corn are the top two most widely grown crops, while in the United States, soybeans and cotton are the two most prevalent GM crops. The majority of GM crops were modified for herbicide tolerance, with smaller percentages modified for insect pest resistance and for both herbicide tolerance and pest tolerance. According to Whitman, "Globally, acreage of GM crops has increased twenty-five-fold in just five years, from approximately 4.3 million acres in 1996 to 109 million acres in 2000.... Approximately 99 million acres were devoted to GM crops in the U.S. and Argentina alone."[21]

There are other foods to watch for and buy only organic. Rice is genetically modified to contain high amounts of vitamin A. Sugar cane is genetically modified to be resistant to certain pesticides. A large percentage of sweeteners used in processed food actually come from corn, not sugar cane or beets. Transgenic papayas now cover about three quarters of the total Hawaiian papaya crop. Meat and dairy products often come from animals that have eaten GM feed, which is why it's very important to only purchase pasture-fed, organically raised animal products. Genetically modified peas have created immune responses in mice, suggesting that they could also create serious allergic reactions in people.[22] The peas had been inserted with a gene from kidney beans, which creates a protein that acts as a pesticide. Many vegetable oils and margarines used in restaurants and in processed foods and salad dressings are made from soy, corn, canola, or cottonseed. Unless these oils specifically say "Non-GMO" or "organic," they are probably genetically modified.

Even vitamin supplements may be genetically modified: Vitamin C is often made from corn, and vitamin E is usually made from soy. Vitamins A, B_2, B_6, B_{12}, D, and K may have fillers derived from GM corn sources, such as starch, glucose, and maltodextrin.[23] This is precisely the reason we should purchase only high-quality vitamins from reliable sources that use organic materials.

Currently, labeling of GMO food is not required; therefore, we must become informed consumers and careful shoppers. We can look at the labels of packaged products to see if they contain corn flour or cornmeal, soy flour, cornstarch, textured vegetable protein, corn syrup, or modified food starch. Check labels of soy sauce, tofu, soy beverages, soy protein isolate, soy milk, soy ice cream, margarine, and soy lecithin, among dozens of other products. If it doesn't say organic or non-GMO for these foods, the chances are strong that they are GMO.

Chapter 3

The Alkalinizing Benefits of the Turbo Diet

YOU JUST DOWNED a sports drink and an energy bar. It seemed like a good choice after a workout, right? However, looking at this combo regarding weight loss and alkaline-acid balance, it's not a great choice. Sports drinks can be among the most acidic of the things we can drink. In fact, these drinks are so acidic they promote tooth erosion. A British dentist analyzed the acidity of eight sports drinks after seeing a twenty-three-year-old runner with severely eroded front teeth who often quenched his thirst with sports drinks. All eight drinks analyzed were below the safe pH of 5.5.[1]

As for the popular energy bar—most energy bars contain a lot of sweetener. It's usually the first or second ingredient in the ingredients label, which means it's loaded with sugar of some type. Sweeteners are acidic. They also set you up for a glycemic response and ultimately insulin resistance. This is just one example of typical American choices that are acidic or turn acidic when digested, thus creating mild acidosis, weight gain, and ill health.

Your body must maintain a delicate, precise pH balance in the blood, which is slightly alkaline. A healthy pH balance in the blood should be between 7.35 and 7.45. To maintain this balance, the body will even draw minerals from bones, teeth, and muscles to use as buffers against the acids.

The acidity or alkalinity of foods can be classified by how we process them. Our bodies transform nearly all foods into acid or alkaline bases. Though we need a balance of different foods for good health, most people eat far more acid-producing foods than alkaline-forming foods. Too many acid-producing substances cause a chronic condition called acidosis, which means the body has become too acidic. Additionally, acid is produced in your body whenever you experience stress or strong emotions. You can see that the typical Western diet and lifestyle move us in the wrong direction. Dr. Robert Young, author of *The pH Miracle for Weight Loss,* has been saying for years that obesity is an acid problem and that fat is saving our lives.[2]

OBESITY IS AN ACID PROBLEM

What happens to your body when you're overly acidic? Acids act on your tissues like meat tenderizer on a New York strip. The body will do whatever it can to protect your delicate tissues and organs from this caustic action. What can't be neutralized is often stored in fat cells to protect vital and more delicate parts. The body will even make more fat cells for storage as needed. That means we could gain more and more weight while not even overeating.

This slightly acidic condition also sets us up for weak bones and teeth. Over time the body will leach calcium from bones and teeth to act as buffers to neutralize acids and maintain the pH balance in the blood. This could account for one reason why osteoporosis is on the rise and why many people shrink in height as they age.

Overacidity also contributes to the deterioration of muscles since magnesium is leached out of muscles to act as a buffer for the acid. This could account for one reason we're seeing a drastic increase in fibromyalgia—a condition characterized by muscle and joint pain that is often helped by magnesium supplementation. That's why juicing magnesium-rich vegetables such as chard, collards, spinach, beet tops, and other hearty greens is very helpful.

If all that is not enough to get your attention, too much acid also contributes to inflammation (a major factor in heart disease), aging (including the skin), and kidney stones. If you want to look younger and prevent diseases caused by inflammation, along with losing weight, it's very wise to eat an alkaline-rich diet like the Turbo Diet.

Most of the foods that make up many slimming diets are acidic. Since eating acid-producing foods piles on the pounds, the solution to being overweight is to cut down on acid-producing foods and eat more alkalinizing foods. And with the alkalinizing effects of fresh juice, your body can let go of fat.

Alkaline Balance Contributes to a Strong Metabolism

Fat cells are much less active than other cells. For example, they burn less energy than muscle cells. The more fat you have relative to muscle, the lower your metabolic rate. But as your body starts burning fat because you are ingesting more alkaline-rich juices and foods, your metabolism will get stronger. You will be able to eat more of the right kinds of foods and still lose weight.

Alkaline balance also contributes to better oxygen transport. The blood plays a very important role in your health—it carries oxygen and nutrients to all the cells. When your blood is optimally pH balanced, it carries oxygen more efficiently. Oxygen contributes to a strong metabolism, gives you energy, and keeps you healthy. It also plays a key role in how well you sleep. Blood cells tend to clump together in a more acidic environment. Healthy red blood cells are spaced apart from each other. Consequently, the blood can move freely throughout the body and get into even the small capillaries. As a result, you feel like your whole body is energized.

During deep sleep, proper blood flow is important for healing and repair. When your blood is healthy, your sleep is energizing and rejuvenating, and you need less of it. Conversely, research confirms that when we don't sleep well, we tend to eat more food, especially the fattening, high-carb (acidic) stuff that packs on the pounds. Also, without ample oxygen, the metabolism slows down and food digests more slowly, causing weight gain, sluggishness, and food fermentation. Fermented food contributes to yeast overgrowth, fungus, and mold throughout the body. These pathogens can cause weight gain and an inability to lose weight. For more information on what to do about yeast overgrowth, see chapter 5.

WHY VEGGIE JUICES AND ALKALINE FOODS FACILITATE WEIGHT LOSS

One important factor of the Turbo Diet is that it is predominantly an alkaline diet. Achieving a 75 percent alkaline to a 25 percent acid balance in foods and beverages and regulating your body's acid/alkaline chemistry through simple dietary changes can result in weight loss, increased energy, and a greater sense of well-being.

Throughout history until the last century, most people's diets were more alkaline than acidic. Because most people couldn't catch or afford to buy a lot of meat, they relied more on vegan foods such as beans and vegetables. Today, people rely heavily on animal products as the main part of their diet. Research shows that a diet high in animal protein produces excess acid, while a diet high in plant foods leaves the body neutral or slightly alkaline. A German study of seven hundred twenty children showed that those eating more fruits and vegetables produced less acid than those eating more meat, dairy, eggs, and grains.[3] Acidic foods and beverages include meat, poultry, eggs, dairy, fish, oxidized oils, trans fats, sweets, sodas, sports drinks, coffee, black tea, alcohol, junk food, and many grains.

Once you stop eating a large quantity of acidic foods and beverages, the body doesn't have to hang on to fat cells as it did before. As the acid/alkaline balance becomes healthier, the body can then haul off a bunch of those little fat storage units. Your metabolism will perk up because your adrenal and thyroid function will improve. Listen up! That happens because too much acid impairs thyroid and adrenal function, meaning there's a drop in the hormones needed for a fired-up metabolism. With slow hormone activity, the body won't turn fat and calories into energy as easily. Many people in this condition say they don't eat a lot of food and should be losing weight, but they just can't seem to drop even a pound or two when they're very strict. I've looked at many dieters' diaries and have found that often people are indeed eating small portions and still not losing weight. Alas, in those cases it's what they're eating rather than the quantity. With an alkalinizing, nutrient-rich diet that helps to get your hormones back in balance, enzyme production and metabolism "get up and going!"

Adding high-alkaline vegetable juices to your diet makes weight loss easier than ever because not only are the juices alkaline, but also they are already broken down and simple to digest. That means they are used quickly to alkalize and energize your body. And they are packed with minerals and other nutrients that help you achieve an acid/alkaline balance without leaching minerals from your bones, teeth, and muscles. And that spells better health in the future.

Nita Lost 42 Pounds

Having gone through a recent divorce and a weight gain of 50 pounds over the past year and a half, I really needed to make a change. In early July 2008 I began to follow Cherie's program by eating only foods from the alkaline food list and avoiding most foods from the acidic list. I also increased my water intake. By the end of July, I had lost 8 pounds just doing this alone. I then began juicing. I also tried a nine-day juice cleanse. I dropped another 12 pounds–totaling 20 pounds in the first month! I ate all organic whole foods, and about 90 percent of that was raw. My energy level increased dramatically, enabling me to start jogging; actually, it was more like "chugging." Then I started Cherie's colon cleanse program and subsequently lost another 20 pounds.

I lost a total of 42 pounds in a mere twelve weeks into my new lifestyle. I started at 168 pounds. I now weigh 126.

I'm an aesthetician and have influenced several of my clients and colleagues at the hotel spa where I work. Many of them are enjoying wonderful results of their own. I feel so good about starting this juicing and healthy lifestyle movement at our downtown spa.

—Nita

NOTE FROM AUTHOR: You can view Nita's before and after pictures at http.//www.juiceladyinfo.com/weightLoss.shtml.

What Is pH?

The pH ranges from 0 to 14, with 7.0 being neutral. Anything above 7.0 is alkaline; anything below 7.0 is considered acidic. The pH is the measurement of the acidity or alkalinity of a solution, which is the actual measurement of hydrogen ions. The letters pH stand for the potential of hydrogen; the H is capitalized because it's the symbol for hydrogen. Increased hydrogen ions (less bonding) result in a drop of the pH (more acidic), while a decrease in hydrogen ions results in a pH rise (more alkaline). The higher the pH reading, the more the solution is alkaline. The lower the pH reading, the more the solution is acidic.

The pH of human blood should be slightly alkaline, between 7.35 and 7.45. The body continually strives to keep this balance. When it's compromised, many problems can occur. Even a slight pH imbalance can make you feel tired, cause you to gain weight, give you trouble digesting food, and contribute to aches and pains in your body. Most

parts of the body have a pH range that differs. The skin can vary from
4.5 to 7.0, for example. Stomach acid ranges vary from 1.0 to 3.0. And
pancreatic secretions can range from 8.0 to 8.3. But the blood is not so
flexible; its range is very narrow. If the pH of your blood goes outside
the range 7.35–7.45 even just a little, your organ function is compromised. If it strays too far from the acceptable range for very long, your
body will go into shock, a coma, and possibly death. That kind of severe
metabolic acidosis is rare; however, mild acidosis is now thought to be
common—affecting at least half of the population.

How to Test Your pH

By analyzing your body's fluids, you can measure what's going on
inside your body. It's a good practice to test either one hour before or
two hours after eating. You can test your urine and saliva with litmus
test strips that are typically sold at drugstores.

Saliva pH test

When you test your saliva, fill your mouth with saliva and then
swallow. This helps remove acidic bacteria. Don't rinse your mouth
before testing the saliva, as this will record the alkalinity of the water
or other liquid you used. Wet a piece of litmus paper with your saliva.
While generally more acidic than blood, salivary pH mirrors the blood.
It is a fair indicator of the extra cellular fluids of your body. Saliva pH
can range anywhere from 5.5 to 7.5 or more. The optimal pH for saliva
is 6.5 to 7.5. A reading lower than 6.5 is indicative of insufficient alkaline reserves. After eating, the saliva pH should rise to 7.5 or above. If
you have enough minerals, your saliva test should register a nice 7.0
to 7.5. If your mineral reserves are too low, you'll typically test 6.4 or
below. Some people test as low as 4.5 to 5.75. (Keep in mind that the
pH scale works like the Richter scale; it's logarithmic. A pH of 5.0 is
one hundred times too acidic.) If your pH tests are that low (acidic),
you should take immediate action to correct the acidity by increasing
your minerals and drinking vegetable juices rich in dark leafy greens
and green stalks such as broccoli, asparagus stems, and broccoli stems
mixed with cucumber, carrot, and lemon (very alkaline).

Urine pH test

When testing your urine, let some urine flow before testing it. This
will give a more accurate reading. The pH of the urine indicates how

the body is working to maintain the proper pH of the blood. The pH of urine points out the efforts of the body to regulate pH through the buffer system. Urine can provide a fairly accurate picture of body chemistry, since values are based on what the body is eliminating. Urine pH can vary from 4.5 to 9.0, but the ideal range is 6.0 to 7.0. If your urinary pH fluctuates from 6.0 to 6.5 first thing in the morning and between 6.5 and 7.0 in the evening before dinner, your body is functioning within a healthy range.

The urine test may indicate how well your body is excreting acids and assimilating minerals, especially calcium, magnesium, sodium, and potassium. These minerals function as buffers. Buffers are substances that help maintain and balance the body against too much acidity or too much alkalinity. If the body's buffering system is over-whelmed, a state of stress exists, and attention should be given right away to reducing the stress through diet and stress reduction. Follow juicing recommendations under the saliva pH test above.

The reason that there is such a difference between your urine and saliva readings is that the mouth is more likely to be acidic. However, when you brush your teeth, the reading will show a high alkaline reading due to the toothpaste. The urine usually shows more of a reflection of the processes the body is undertaking to remove acid from the body.

Someone who eats a typical American diet would be more likely to have a saliva pH average of about 5.5–6.0. This may not seem much lower than the normal range; however, it is important to remember, as mentioned earlier, that the pH scale is logarithmic; each step is ten times the previous step. For example, 5.5 is one hundred times more acidic than 6.5.

Testing the pH of your saliva or urine is only going to give you a general trend. Unfortunately, there is no way of determining the exact pH of the blood without undergoing a live blood analysis.

How the Acidic/Alkaline Value of Food Is Determined

Acidic/alkaline diet food chart quantifications come from the pH of the ash that results from the body burning food for fuel. The alkaline/acidic value is determined by measuring unused minerals. When we digest a food, it produces a residue. That's how we classify it as an alkaline or acidic food. When we digest a food, it is chemically oxidized (burned) to form water, carbon dioxide, and an inorganic compound. The alkaline or acidic nature of the inorganic compound formed determines whether the food is alkaline or acidic. If it contains more sodium, potassium, or calcium, it's classed as an alkaline food. If it contains more sulfur, phosphate, or chloride, it's classed as an acidic food.

There are inconsistencies between the acid- or alkaline-forming values given in the lists provided by health writers and researchers, and very few reliable references. A number of practitioners go by personal experience with clients, measurements with litmus paper, and health results gathered over time because that's the only thing available.

Regardless of a lack of research, the principles are clear—drink plenty of vegetable juices; eat lots of vegetables, sprouts, fruit, nuts, and seeds; and eat sparingly acid-producing foods such as dairy products, grains, and protein from eggs, poultry, meat, and fish. But remember, you don't have to cut out all acid-forming foods—eating some is necessary for health. It's recommended that no more than about 25 percent of our diet comes from the acidic category and the remaining 75 percent from alkaline foods. This will probably mean you need to shift the overall balance of your diet toward vegan foods (the alkaline group) and away from the excessively acid-forming diet of a quick-food culture.

Acidic and Alkaline Foods

Most health professionals agree that this list is fairly accurate when it comes to alkaline and acidic foods.

Acidic Foods	Alkaline Foods
Meat	Vegetable juices
Poultry	Vegetables
Eggs	Sprouts
Dairy	Fruit
Fish	Seeds and nuts
Grains	Legumes (beans, lentils, split peas)
Trans fats	Healthy oils such as coconut and olive
Sugar and sweets	

Acidic Foods	Alkaline Foods
Sodas	
Sports drinks	
Coffee	
Black tea	
Alcohol (wine, beer, liquor)	
Junk food	

FOOD COMBINING AND DIGESTION

Ivan Pavlov, famous for his research with dogs, proved that the digestive enzymes released and the amount of acid secreted depend on the type of food we eat. His experiments showed that starches and proteins, when eaten separately, are digested in just a few hours, but a protein-starch mixture could still be digesting many hours later. He also showed that when foods are eaten before the digestion of one mixture has been completed, fermentation may develop.[4] For example, when fruit is eaten shortly after a meal, many people say that it gives them gas.

The enzymes essential for digestion function at specific pH levels. Protein and carbohydrate enzymes each require different pH levels. If you mix them together in the "same bag," you won't be able to digest either food well. If you put fresh fruit on top of a big meal, it has to sit around waiting until the other food is digested, during which time bacteria attack the fruit and ferment it, gobbling up nutrients and producing gas and metabolic wastes.

How does food combining play out in our daily life? Want to try an experiment? Eat a steak or piece of chicken and potatoes for lunch, and then monitor how you feel about an hour after the meal. The next day eat a steak or piece of chicken with a large green salad but no potatoes, pasta, or bread. Which day did you feel more drowsy or alert? Sluggish or energized? The worst combinations of foods are animal proteins and starches like bread, pasta, pizza, or potatoes. This is a significant setup for weight gain. And it's a typical American meal. If you never follow any other rule of food combining, try omitting the starch-protein combination from your diet.

Dr. Hay's Experiment

In 1908 after practicing medicine for sixteen years, Dr. William Howard Hay developed Bright's disease (kidney disease), high blood pressure, and a dilated heart. Since there was no treatment available, Dr. Hay decided to cure himself. He looked at the process of digestion, the enzymes that are essential for this process, and whether the food has an overall acidifying or alkalinizing effect on the body. Through changing his diet, Dr. Hay totally astounded his colleagues with a complete remission of his symptoms and diseases. He also reduced his weight by about 45 pounds. In 1911 he introduced food-combining guidelines, the Hay Diet, emphasizing the need to combine foods properly and reduce acidifying foods.[5]

An Alkaline-Rich Diet Helps Prevent Osteoporosis

Osteoporosis is a major health concern for an estimated 44 million people, affecting 55 percent of our population over fifty years old. We seem to know more about this disease today than at any other time in history. We choke down calcium pills and eat dairy products because we're told they're good sources of calcium, and we exercise to strengthen our bones as well as our muscles. But alas! Our bones are getting worse, per capita, than ever before. Why is that?

A study on cola beverage consumption with rats showed detrimental effects on bone density. The rats were fed colas and the effects on bone density were measured. The study suggests that colas have the potential of reducing bone density because they contribute to a depletion of minerals.[6]

When you eat too many acid-forming foods, calcium is leached from the bones, say Tufts University researchers. They found that taking an alkaline supplement actually reduced calcium loss by 20 percent.[7] Though the supplement is not available at the time of this writing, you can get great alkalinizing benefits by vegetable juicing, taking a mineral supplement, and making sure that you get six to nine servings of fruits and vegetables each day. Additionally, you will benefit by cutting back on acid-producing foods. *The Juice Lady's Turbo Diet* outlines a great plan to help you prevent this bone-weakening disease.

Science in Support of an Alkaline Diet

A study at the University of California discovered that as we grow older, beginning around age forty-five, we start losing some of the alkaline buffer bicarbonates in our blood. This study has shown that acid-producing diets do indeed produce a low-grade systemic acidosis in otherwise healthy adult subjects. And the degree of acidosis increases with age.[8]

The *American Journal of Clinical Nutrition* concluded that alkalinizing diets improve bone density and growth hormone concentrations, whereas acidic diets contribute to bone and muscle loss.[9] In a study at the University of Chicago, participants consumed a low-carbohydrate, high-protein diet for six weeks. They all produced more acid in their urine and showed signs of increased kidney stone formation and bone loss.[10]

In his book *Reverse Aging*, Dr. Sang Whang suggests that we age because we gradually accumulate acidic wastes.[11] These wastes show up as uric acid, urate, sulfate, phosphate, kidney stones, and other organic wastes. Cellulite is pockets of these trapped toxins and acidic wastes stored in fat and water below the skin.

Addressing the Opposition

You should know that not all health professionals believe there is any benefit in eating more alkaline foods than acid-producing foods. They point out that everything is acidic in the stomach and becomes alkaline in the intestinal tract due to pancreatic secretions. The blood pH range is so narrow that any measurable change would cause death. Even a bottle of antacids won't affect the acidity of the stomach for long, they say.

Though these scientific facts are true, it doesn't mean that the body isn't affected by excess acid-forming foods. The body may correct the pH of the blood, while tissues, bones, teeth, and muscles are sacrificing themselves to keep the blood normal.

Let's take a look at what happens when you drink soda. A 350-milliliter serving of Coke, Pepsi, or similar soft drink delivers between 9 and 11 teaspoons of sugar. This, along with other components of soda, is so acidic that the body must react swiftly by drawing large amounts of calcium and magnesium from the body's stores, which can come from bones, teeth, and muscles, pouring it into the system to neutralize the excess acid to quickly restore balance.

A typical American diet high in acid-producing foods places pressure on the body's regulating systems to maintain pH stability. The extra buffering required can deplete the body of important minerals such as sodium, potassium, magnesium, and calcium. Minerals are often borrowed from vital organs, bones, muscles, and teeth to buffer (neutralize) the acid. This presents a problem. Keeping the body at a normal or near-normal pH means the buffer systems are being taxed, which puts a strain on the whole system. The typical American diet particularly plays havoc with tissues, joints, and organs of the body.

Chef Mia's Weight-Loss Journey

My driver's license said I weighed 198 pounds, but actually I was over 200 pounds. I just couldn't face being that heavy without the excuse of being pregnant. With each of my two children I had gained about 50 pounds but lost it within a year or two after their births. This time was different. My weight gain seemed to go hand in hand with the depression, chronic fatigue, and neurological problems associated with a traumatic brain injury I'd sustained. It wasn't easy for me to just pick myself up off the couch and get moving after the accident. I had no energy. An exercise routine, even walking, was neurologically overstimulating and left me so cognitively and physically exhausted that it took hours and sometimes days to recover. I couldn't move enough for a workout.

Since being hit by a car while riding my bicycle, I'd spent most of my time on the couch or in bed and always in pain. Unsolicited advice from a well-meaning neighbor who saw me grow from the slender 145-pound person I'd been to over 200 pounds had me questioning my food choices and my inability to figure out how to "keep moving and stop eating."

Then I discovered raw vegan cuisine and juicing by reading various authors in the field of juicing, raw vegan cuisine, and nutrition. In each book I marveled at the consistent case studies and personal reports from people who experienced weight loss and healing with juicing and eating lots of raw foods. As I read the books and looked at before and after pictures with each person radiating an inescapable beauty that shone through their eyes, I learned about their relief from physical symptoms and weight loss— from a few pounds to several hundred. I experienced hope. All the healings and weight-loss stories took place through a simple act of eating. I began to realize that at the very least, losing 50 pounds could become a reality.

In the first year I drank a lot of wheatgrass juice. A few weeks into my new program, I went for my usual dental checkup and cleaning. My hygienist asked if I had whitened my teeth and marveled at the plasticity of my previously receding gum line. Now, healthy toned gums hugged my teeth. She thought I had just come back from a sunny vacation somewhere because my skin glowed and appeared tanned, but I assured her I had not been anywhere. She commented that I was talking faster and appeared to understand her, and she didn't have to repeat things to me so much on this visit. She has watched me transform over the years and continues to marvel at the changes. "It's like you're a totally different person!" she recently said.

My dietary program paid off. I lost more than I expected– about 70 pounds in seven months. I've been eating a high raw-food diet for about four years and have kept the weight off, fluctuating between 134–142 pounds.

—CHEF MIA

THE TURBO DIET SUPPORTS WEIGHT LOSS ALONG WITH WELLNESS

Unless your body's pH level is slightly alkaline, you won't experience weight loss, good health, or healing if you're ill. So no matter what means you choose to get rid of excess weight or improve your health, it won't be truly effective until your body's pH level is balanced. If your body remains slightly acidic, it's going to hold on to fat cells for the sake of your life.

And you won't be able to effectively assimilate vitamins or minerals. Acidosis will decrease your body's ability to absorb minerals and other nutrients, decrease the energy production in the cells, and decrease its ability to repair damaged cells. It will decrease the ability to detoxify heavy metals. It will also create an environment for tumor cells to thrive. And it can cause fatigue and illness.

An acid-forming diet, emotional stress, toxic overload, immune reactions, or any process depriving the cells of oxygen and nutrients can cause acidic pH. The body will try to compensate by utilizing minerals as a buffer. But if the body doesn't get enough minerals from the diet to bring the pH into balance, an acidic buildup occurs. And when the acid overload gets too high, excess acid is dumped into the cells in order to maintain balance.

Acidosis can cause such problems as:

- Weight gain or obesity
- Diabetes
- Cardiovascular damage
- Bladder conditions
- Kidney stones
- Immune deficiency
- Free-radical damage
- Hormonal problems
- Premature aging
- Osteoporosis and joint pain
- Aching muscles and lactic acid buildup
- Low energy and chronic fatigue
- Slow digestion and elimination
- Yeast/fungal overgrowth
- Lower body temperature
- Frequent infections
- Loss of joy and enthusiasm
- Depression
- Being easily stressed
- Pale complexion
- Headaches
- Inflammation of the cornea and eyelids
- Inflamed, sensitive gums
- Mouth and stomach ulcers
- Cracks at the corners of the lips
- Excess stomach acid
- Gastritis
- Nails that are thin and split easily
- Dull hair, split ends, hair falling out
- Dry skin
- Skin irritation
- Leg cramps and spasms

As you balance protein with plenty of alkaline-rich vegetables and vegetable juices and complement your diet with greens and mineral supplements, you should achieve alkaline balance in your body and prevent acid buildup. This will help to prevent bone loss, muscle deterioration, and many other ailments associated with mild acidosis. And it will help you achieve the weight you desire and want to maintain.

Chapter 4

The Turbo Diet Exercise Plan

Have you always wished you had the energy to exercise? Now that you're juicing and eating more alkaline-rich foods, you should have the energy it takes to get up and go. Exercise is an important step in the weight-loss process. Think of this step as enjoyable movement rather than a chore. Movement is a key word, because your body was made to be in motion. It was marvelously fashioned to walk, run, swim, dance, jog, lift, jump, bend, stretch, work, and play. A healthy, trim, energetic, and vibrant body is a body that moves.

For many people, the natural inclination of the body to move has been lost through years of inactivity—too many of us sit in one position all day long. We begin to think of the joy of movement as the *work* of exercise. Often, we don't do enough exercising because we're tired from the stresses of daily life, especially the pressures of work and home, along with not having enough live, energizing food in our diet to give us the power we need to get moving.

The good news is that even a small amount of exercise done consistently over time produces big rewards. You will not only look and feel better, but you will also be nourished and strengthened—inside and out.

Movement builds strong muscles, bones, and connective tissue. And exercise creates a body that is trim and fit. Exercise also has numerous benefits for your internal body. It strengthens the immune system, keeps your heart and cardiovascular system healthy, helps metabolize nutrients, builds new proteins and hormones, carries waste products out of your system, relieves stress, boosts growth hormones (which helps build muscles), promotes restful, peaceful sleep, and, of course, burns calories.

Ask just about any exercise physiologist, physical therapist, or anyone else in the health field for that matter, and they will tell you that exercise is an important part of a weight-loss plan. If you're physically able, even a slight increase in your level of activity will help you feel better, sleep better, and lose weight, with particularly noticeable benefits if you've been leading a sedentary lifestyle. Just half an hour of moderate exercise, like walking, can be enough to help you improve your physical fitness and facilitate your weight loss.

IT'S TIME TO GET GOING!

There are scores of different ways to exercise to lose weight and feel great. Maybe you already have a favorite way of exercising, but perhaps you will be inspired to try something new you haven't tried before after finishing this chapter. Different movements are designed to achieve diverse results. The following suggestions are divided into three general categories: aerobic exercises, weight and resistance training, and strengthening and stretching exercises. For a balanced routine, choose something from each category. Your initial goal should be to exercise three or more times throughout the week for about forty-five to sixty minutes at a time. The most important factor is to be consistent.

What to Do If You Have Physical Limitations

Consider using a rebounder, a lymphasizer, or a swimming pool if you have physical limitations or disabilities. For my recommendations of specific products, see Appendix A.

AEROBIC EXERCISES

Aerobic literally means *in the presence of oxygen*. Our bodies require oxygen in each cell for the production of energy. Aerobic activities are those that bring maximum energy into our cells through sustained activities that rely on oxygen for energy. These activities build endurance, burn fat, and condition the cardiovascular system.

You could begin with thirty to sixty minutes three or four times a week. Thirty minutes would be good for those who have been inactive or who are just beginning to exercise. As you progress in your exercise regimen, you will probably want to increase the time and intensity of your workouts, perhaps adding a few different activities that are highlighted in this chapter. Go slowly at first, and remember it is consistent exercise over time that yields the most benefits. Check with your doctor if you have any health concerns, and then get going!

Aerobic exercise is an ideal way to dissipate the excess energy that builds up with a high-stress lifestyle or simply sitting too much. Rather than eating more food, drinking more coffee, taking drugs, or snapping at the kids, spouse, or co-workers, why not take an exercise break? It's healthier and far more effective to channel pent-up emotions and excess energy into an active form of working out.

Aerobic activities like walking, jogging, swimming, bicycling, racquet sports, skiing, step aerobics classes, and dancing are great for weight loss. Find something you enjoy so your exercise is fun; otherwise, you probably won't stick with it. There are a number of possibilities listed in the pages that follow, but there are certainly many other activities that aren't discussed here. And do what you can to get a bit of exercise every day, even if it's parking farther away from the entrance at work or taking the stairs instead of the elevator. You will build muscles and rev up your metabolism so that you'll burn more calories, even at a resting heart rate; thus helping to lose weight, look more toned, and feel more energized.

Cycling

Cycling is an excellent aerobic conditioner if it's done with enough intensity and for a sufficient time. Just coasting around the neighborhood on your bicycle will not get your heart rate up. But sustained cycling will build strength, increase endurance, and help reduce stress. Depending on the speed and terrain, you can burn 350 to 450 calories or more an hour.

Cycling is sought after because it produces less stress on the body than running. It's also an excellent choice for anyone who is unable to run or do other activities like step aerobics because of orthopedic problems, conditions that are aggravated by weight-bearing exercises, or being overweight.

Outdoor biking is fun in the summer or in warmer climates but not when the weather is bad. The alternative for biking enthusiasts is the indoor stationary bike that can keep you just as fit. Most health clubs have stationery bikes and cycling classes, which increase motivation for most people.

Fast walking, jogging, and running

Fast walking, jogging, or running is a great aerobic movement you can do almost anywhere or anytime. The idea is to get your heart working hard enough to boost you to greater cardiovascular fitness. Gradually increasing the intensity of your workout by speeding up your pace will help you to lose weight more quickly and push your body out of its comfort zone. Try increasing your pace until you are uncomfortable for a minute, then fall back to your normal stride. Fast walking, jogging, or running can be done outside or inside on a treadmill. One advantage of the treadmill is that you can increase the incline so you burn more calories while maintaining the same pace.

Fast walking puts less stress on your body than running, especially your knees and ankles. If you move fast enough and go far enough—five miles an hour for forty-five minutes or more—it can get you just as fit as running or jogging. If you have the time, walking at slower speeds for an hour or more will help you burn the maximum amount of fat. High-energy walking styles, like race walking, are better than running for building strength in your arms and torso and streamlining flabby thighs.

Running has other benefits such as the "runner's high," which results from the release of endorphins, the body's "feel-good" brain neurotransmitters that have pain-relieving properties.

Fast walking, jogging, or running with consistency has been shown to prevent muscle and bone loss that often occurs with age. Our bones are made for movement. By sitting at a desk or computer all day and getting very little exercise in our free time, our bones can grow weaker. However, by fast walking or jogging regularly, the frame gets the demands it needs to stay healthy. In addition to keeping our bones and internal organs from aging quickly, regular, high-intensity exercise, like fast walking and running, has also been proven to promote the release of the human growth hormone (HGH), which promotes weight loss and better sleep.

During aerobic activity your arteries expand and contract nearly three times as much as usual. Fast walking, jogging, or running helps to strengthen the heart muscle, maintain the elasticity of the arteries, and lower blood pressure, thus reducing the risk of hypertension, stroke, and heart attack. These activities also raise HDL (the "good" cholesterol), reduce the risk of blood clots, and encourage the use of part of your lungs that usually go unused. Additionally, they boost the immune system by creating a higher concentration of lymphocytes, which are the white blood cells that attack infection, bacteria, and viruses.

Rebounding

Rebounding is an exercise performed on a mini-trampoline known as a rebounder. This workout is fun, easy to do, safe, and can be done in your own home. There's no need to pound the pavement, dodge cars, or put up with bad weather. Rebounding is a zero-impact, aerobic exercise that improves circulation and increases the capacity of both the heart and lungs. With regular rebounding, your resting heart rate can decline on average about ten beats per minute.

Rebounding protects the joints from damage. Unlike jogging on hard surfaces, which puts lots of stress on joints such as the ankles and knees and can damage them, rebounding affects joints, tendons, and muscles equally.

The body has no active lymph pump to move lymph through the vessels the way our heart pumps blood through the blood vessels. The lymph system is passive, and it has valves that move it in only one direction. Therefore, active movement is required to keep lymph fluids moving. The main lymphatic vessels run up the legs, arms, and torso, so the vertical up-and-down movement of rebounding is very effective at pumping the lymph.

The lymphatic system cannot properly excrete toxic wastes without adequate movement. One of the best advantages of rebounding is that it helps the lymphatic system move waste out of the body. When the lymph is not moved along through adequate exercise, it can cause us to feel out of sorts and tired.

Rebounding has many other health-enhancing benefits. For example, it is good for promoting deep relaxation. It helps manage body composition and improves muscle-to-fat ratio. It improves metabolic rate so that more calories are burned even after exercise. It circulates oxygen to the tissues and organs and helps move fluids through the body. It strengthens the heart and other muscles in the body so that they work more efficiently. It also helps to lower circulating cholesterol and triglyceride levels and improves digestion and elimination.

The best way to begin rebounding is to bounce slowly, keeping your feet in contact with the rebounder's surface as your body moves up and down. This gentle movement will strengthen your body. As your strength and balance increase, you can bounce higher and faster.

It's fun to listen to music while you bounce, but you can also watch television or listen to your favorite radio show as you bounce away on your rebounder.

You can wear running shoes or jump with bare feet; just make sure that there's nothing on your feet to make you slip, such as socks. Start with five to ten minutes and increase your time as your fitness improves. If you're older or have been inactive for a while, start with just a few minutes and work up. It's important to gradually build up your time, especially if you're out of shape.

The rebounder is ideal to use if you have physical limitations. If you have joint or knee problems and have not been able to exercise, you may find that rebounding gives you a way to get moving. Blind or handicapped people can purchase a handrail that attaches to the rebounder.

An Exercise Machine for Everyone: The Lymphasizer (Swing Machine)

The lymphasizer, also known as the healthy swinger or swing machine, is an ideal alternative or a great addition to an exercise regimen because it will actively move the lymph and blood through the body when you lie down on the floor with your feet in the grooves of the machine. It's very beneficial for those who have circulation problems in their feet stemming from such things as diabetes or steroid drug use. With this machine, you will have a zero-impact workout that requires no active movement. You just lie on the floor with your feet on the machine and get the aerobic benefits of a half hour of exercise in about ten to fifteen minutes.

The lymphasizer provides a simple exercise without applying any stress on the spine, ankles, knees, or other body parts. Simply lie on the floor, and it will rock your body from side to side like the movement of a fish. This simple rocking motion maintains a proper energy balance and oxygen supply to the body. Regular use of this relaxing massage movement stimulates your body and achieves relaxation and stress reduction. A sense of well-being arises from the massaging, swing action that is immediately noticeable. Using the lymphasizer before bedtime promotes more restful sleep as well as weight loss.

Though this machine is a great addition for everyone, it can be excellent for the disabled, for anyone with serious knee or ankle problems, for those who are very overweight and find other forms of exercise difficult, or for those who for other medical reasons are unable to even bounce slowly on a rebounder. (For more information on the lymphasizer, see Appendix A.)

Step and dance aerobics

Put on your step shoes and get ready to move to the music. Step aerobics is fun and a great workout. You may be like me and many other people who enjoy working out with others in a class setting. I think it's more motivating, fun, and encouraging to work out with other people than to work out alone. Plus, with a class you have a set time when you have to show up for a class, which is more motivating for some than a self-determined schedule. Almost every gym and health club has several aerobics classes to choose from—step aerobics, nonstep aerobics, dance aerobics classes, and total body workouts that combine light weights with step for lots of movement, muscle building, and aerobic benefit. Find a class that you like and go for it! Total body workout is one of my favorites.

Swimming

Swimming tones your entire body while providing an excellent cardiovascular workout. It strengthens your heart muscle and improves delivery of oxygen to your muscles. It's hard to beat when it comes to a sport that builds the body, soothes the mind, regulates breathing, stimulates circulation, and puts no stress on the joints. It's an ideal exercise for just about everyone—old; young; overweight; people with hip, knee, and ankle problems; and active people with no health problems at all. Plus, swimming has a calorie-burning potential of 350 to 420 calories per hour, so it's great for weight loss. The obvious disadvantage is that you need a pool, which is not always an option.

You can begin by holding on to the side of the pool and kicking or moving your arms and legs. Another suggestion is to simply walk slowly back and forth across the shallow end of the pool. The increased resistance of the water will help to strengthen the muscles without putting strain on joints and ligaments.

Water aerobics

Water aerobic workouts usually combine a variety of techniques from land aerobics, including walking or running backward and forward, jumping jacks, mimicking cross-country skiing, along with various arm movements. The workout also may incorporate equipment such as flotation belts, specialized water aerobics shoes, flotation devices, and ankle and wrist weights. The exercise is often done with music in water tempo.

In addition to the standard benefits of other exercise, the use of water supports the body and reduces the risk of muscle or joint injury. The lessening of gravity by flotation places less stress on the joints and can allow a greater range of motion. The easing of gravity also makes water aerobics safe for everyone, including the elderly. Exercise in water can also prevent overheating through continuous cooling of the body. Most water aerobic classes last from forty-five to sixty minutes.

Zumba dance

The Zumba dance workout program is becoming very popular, fusing Latin rhythms and easy-to-follow moves to create a one-of-a-kind fitness program that's more like a dance party than a workout. Zumba offers participants an absolute blast in an exciting hour of calorie-burning, energizing dance movements. The routines feature interval-training sessions where fast and slow rhythms and resistance training are combined to tone and sculpt your body while burning fat. Add some Latin flavor and international music into the mix, and you have a Zumba class. Should you think you might not get a good workout, just go check out a class at your local club. I did. I worked so hard I was dripping by the end of the class—but with a big smile on my face.

Walking

Walking is an exercise that practically anyone can do. You can stroll or fast walk almost anywhere, including indoors, and you'll be burning calories as you go. Walking at a brisk pace will keep you in the midrange of aerobic activity and won't put a strain on your joints and ligaments like some more vigorous forms of aerobic activity.

Walking increases your sense of well-being and gets you outside in the fresh air. Some of the benefits of walking include reduced stress, relaxation of tight muscles, mood elevation, and lessening the symptoms of depression and anxiety. It's something you can do in the evening after dinner to help you sleep better.

The following ideas could help you get going with a consistent walking program:

- Take a short walk before or after dinner to relax your nervous system and at the same time burn calories.
- Find a friend to walk with for companionship and motivation. Dogs are great walking partners too. If you don't have a dog to walk, perhaps you could walk the neighbor's furry friend. Your canine buddy will keep you moving and help you focus on the simple things of life. I can vouch for that! I walk Annie the Schnauzer every morning in addition to my workout classes two to three times a week. Not only have I noticed firmer thighs since we adopted her, but I've also noticed the subtle little things in the neighborhood like the neighbor who sets out a water bowl for dogs every day and the little dog that watches for us inside his fence.
- Walk briskly enough to break a sweat, but not so fast that you run out of breath. Begin to slow down toward the end of your walk to bring your heartbeat down to its resting rate.

WEIGHT AND RESISTANCE TRAINING

Weight-bearing exercises such as strength training with machines and/or free weights are one of the most efficient ways to develop muscle strength and tone. This form of exercise increases lean body mass, which is important for individuals attempting weight loss. Weight training forces your body to produce more muscle, which increases the size and number of mitochondria. Mitochondria are cell organelles that burn glucose and produce energy. They are found in high concentration in heart and skeletal muscles. They can be called cellular furnaces, because this is where nutrients from the food we eat are burned to produce ATP, which produces cellular energy. (ATP is a nucleotide derived from adenosine that occurs in muscle tissue, the major source of energy for cellular reactions.)

Weight and resistance training builds up the bones and connective tissues, thus helping to prevent injuries and osteoporosis. This type of exercise also helps you to develop coordination and balance.

It increases strength, builds and tones muscles, and increases endurance. Weight training also helps you develop self-confidence and body satisfaction because you will look more toned and leaner after only a few short weeks of a concentrated weight-training program.

Weight training counteracts the natural tendency of the body to grow weaker as we age. Weight-bearing exercise is an important component in osteoporosis prevention. Without regular strength training, we can lose up to half a pound of muscle every year after age thirty-five.[1] With weight training, we can stay stronger longer. If you've ever been to a gym with serious weight-training programs, you will see men and women in their fifties, sixties, seventies, and sometimes eighties who look as trim and fit as a thirty- or forty-year-old. This should encourage you to add some form of strength training to your regular routine.

You can boost your strength and improve your appearance no matter how old, weak, or out of shape you are. People over fifty who have not been active or have high blood pressure, heart disease, back pain, arthritis, or any other health problem will want to check with their doctor before beginning any kind of strength-training program.

STRETCHING, RELAXATION, AND BREATHING EXERCISES

Throughout history, many societies have devised exercises that are designed to strengthen and stretch the body while relaxing and focusing the mind. Some of these techniques have elaborate philosophies associated with them, yet the simple essence of their techniques is to stretch and relax the muscles, plus control breathing, so that more oxygen is delivered into the cells, especially the brain, thus calming and relaxing the whole body.

Stretching and relaxation exercises can increase suppleness, enhance mental and physical relaxation, and improve the quality of your sleep. Stretching is something nearly everyone can do, no matter what age or level of ability. Gentle movements, deep breathing, and long stretches are ideal methods of increasing flexibility and relaxation. The advantage of stretching is that it strengthens the nervous system and relieves stress and anxiety. It also strengthens and relaxes the skeletal, muscular, digestive, cardiovascular, and glandular systems, thus helping to calm the body and mind. The body is not overstimulated, as with more strenuous exercise, making this a good choice toward the end of the day.

Pilates

Pilates, a series of exercises designed to improve flexibility and strength through a variety of stretching and balancing movements, has become increasingly popular in the last several years. It typically gives people a longer, leaner appearance. It was developed by Joseph Pilates, a prisoner of war during World War II. Pilates introduced his exercises, which included mat workouts, to inmates in a German internment camp, helping them keep physically fit.

Today, Pilates exercise has become particularly popular among dancers, athletes, celebrities, and models because in addition to helping to develop flexibility without causing a strain on the muscles, it also helps improve posture. A regular Pilates regimen results in a flatter stomach, thinner waist, and leaner thighs, as well as increased mobility in joints. Pilates helps improve strength, tone, flexibility, and balance, and makes the body less prone to injury. It reduces stress, relieves tension, and boosts energy through deep stretching. It also strengthens the back and spine. Physiotherapists recommend Pilates to those seeking rehabilitation after injuries to their limbs. Pilates is recommended for everyone—young, elderly, sedentary, those who suffer from osteoporosis, and those who are overweight.

Chapter 5

Troubleshooting: What to Do When You Don't Lose Weight

I F YOU'VE TRIED to lose weight and just can't seem to get the scale to budge in spite of your best efforts, or you've reached a weight-loss plateau, you may need a specific intervention that gets to the root of why you aren't losing the weight you want to lose. The good news is that when you correct the issue, you will get healthier, and weight loss may end up being a secondary benefit compared to all the other payoffs.

There are numerous reasons why people can't lose weight that go beyond simply eating too many calories and not exercising enough. Are you one of those people who eat very little compared to other people in your life, and still the weight hangs on like gum on your shoe? If you said yes, this chapter is for you. It can help you identify what may be going on in your body that keeps you from enjoying the weight-loss success so many other people have benefited from on the Turbo Diet.

Nancy Overcame Weight-Loss Obstacles and Lost 25 Pounds

I've lost about 25 pounds since I started my juicing, raw foods diet, and cleanse program from Cherie's books. A year before, I'd set a goal to lose 12 pounds and just couldn't do it. Then I went on the juicing, raw foods, and cleanse programs to focus on optimum health because I was diagnosed with breast cancer. Surprisingly, the weight just fell off! I eat a lot of food—all good food, and a high percentage of it is raw. I'm not hungry at all. I have lots of energy. But the best news is that I was able to go through cancer treatments with energy and stamina.

—NANCY

Why Some People Can't Lose Weight No Matter What They Do

Though the Turbo Diet works for most people, there are individuals who have certain health conditions or lifestyle issues that make it very difficult to lose weight. If you are one of those folks, unless the underlying challenge is addressed, you could spend a lifetime pursuing weight loss unsuccessfully. Often when problems are corrected that cause both ill health and weight gain, the weight just melts away naturally. As you heal your body, balance your hormones, detoxify your organs of elimination, identify and eliminate foods that pack on the pounds, and creatively deal with emotional eating, you can achieve and maintain a healthy weight for life.

The late Dr. Robert C. Atkins said that about 20 percent of the people on the Atkins diet didn't lose weight because of a yeast overgrowth known as *Candida albicans*.[1] Candidiasis, as it's also called, is one of the conditions that is covered in this chapter, along with metabolic syndrome, chronic fatigue syndrome, fibromyalgia, low thyroid, sleep disorders, digestive disorders (including irritable bowel syndrome, leaky gut syndrome, Crohn's disease, and colitis), food sensitivities, and stress. I encourage you to read through this chapter even if you don't think anything applies to you. You may be surprised as to what you learn about your body.

Metabolic Syndrome

Although Gerald Reaven, MD, professor emeritus at Stanford University School of Medicine, first identified metabolic syndrome in 1998, its principal component of obesity was not initially emphasized as it is today. Metabolic syndrome, which was discussed in chapter 1, is a combination of obesity, hypercholesterolemia, and hypertension linked by an underlying insulin resistance. Any three of the following traits in any individual signify metabolic syndrome:

- Abdominal obesity: a waist circumference over 102 centimeters (40 inches) in men and over 88 centimeters (35 inches) in women
- High serum triglycerides: 150 mg/dl or above
- Low HDL cholesterol: 40 mg/dl or lower in men and 50 mg/dl or lower in women

- High blood pressure: 130/85 or higher
- High blood sugar: a fasting blood glucose of 110 mg/dl or above (some groups say 100 mg/dl)

Metabolic syndrome is also associated with excess insulin secretion. Excessive dietary intake of sugar and refined flour products, lack of exercise, and genetic tendencies contribute to insulin resistance and the other characteristics that lead to metabolic syndrome. Insulin signals the cells to absorb glucose from the bloodstream. The body monitors the food we've digested, our blood sugar levels, and our cell demands; it then should release insulin in the right amounts for our needs. A healthy body is insulin sensitive, not resistant.

Today most of the calories in an average American diet come from carbohydrates, with many of those being simple carbohydrates—sugars in the form of sweets and refined flour—that quickly enter the bloodstream. The body has to release high levels of insulin to keep the level of glucose in the bloodstream from spiraling out of control. Letting your blood sugar get too high is simply not acceptable. The resulting excess of insulin in the bloodstream is called hyperinsulinemia. The body wasn't designed for prolonged high levels of insulin; it disrupts cellular metabolism and spreads inflammation. Over time the cells quit responding to this signal, and the body becomes insulin resistant. It's like knocking on a door and no one answers anymore.

Insulin resistance causes weight gain because it disrupts fat metabolism. When the cells won't absorb the extra glucose circulating in the bloodstream, the liver converts it into fat. And guess what? Normal fat cells are loaded with glucose receptors that are sensitive to insulin signals. So while the fat cells are gobbling up glucose, the other cells are actually "starved" for glucose. This person feels tired a lot and tends to eat more carbohydrate-rich foods trying to boost energy, which makes her situation even worse. It becomes a frustrating cycle.

The lifestyle changes that turn this syndrome around start with a low-glycemic diet and avoidance of *all* sugar. The Turbo Diet is an ideal plan. On this diet the emphasis is on vegetable juices and lots of vegetables and alkaline-rich foods. You should eliminate sugar and even reduce fruit, eating only low-sugar fruit like a green apple or berries, and avoid all fruit juice except for lemon and lime. Sweeteners, no matter what we call them, are still sugars. Most natural sweeteners such as honey, agave syrup, and pure maple sugar are a little better than refined sugars, in that they have some nutrients and aren't bleached and refined; however, they are still sugar. In addition, you should avoid caffeine and tobacco. Include plenty of healthy fats, especially the omega-3 fats, and avoid animal fats. Limit your salt intake, using only Celtic sea salt, and make sure you exercise at least three to four times per week. All this should help your cells become more responsive to insulin and curb overproduction of insulin. Weight loss should follow without a lot of effort. But the best news is that your health will improve immensely.

Can Diet Sodas Make You Fat?

You put a packet of Splenda in your tea or coffee and feel good about all the calories you saved. You order a diet soda because you don't want to gain weight from sugar-laden sodas. And you buy sugar-free cookies for the same reason. But you notice that you aren't losing weight. Do diet sweeteners really help you keep the weight off? Not according to a Purdue University study released in the journal *Behavioral Neuroscience*. It reported that rats on diets containing the artificial sweetener saccharin gained more weight than rats given sugar-sweetened food. Researchers believe that diet sweeteners change brain chemistry and alter metabolism.[2] And studies have found that diet sweeteners also increase your chance for developing metabolic syndrome.

One study published in the *International Journal of Obesity* (January, 1997), monitored fourteen women on weight-loss diets who were given drinks of aspartame-sweetened lemonade, sucrose-sweetened lemonade, and carbonated mineral water on three separate days. The women ate significantly more food when they drank the aspartame-sweetened beverages.[3] In fact, the University of Texas Health Sciences Center reported a "41% increase in risk of being overweight for every can or bottle of diet soft drink a person consumes each day." The findings come from eight years of collecting data.[4]

A study with animals published in the *Journal of Toxicology and Environmental Health* found that Splenda reduced the amount of good bacteria in the intestines by 50 percent, increased the pH level in the intestines, and contributed to increases in body weight.[5]

Alas, as you can see, there isn't one good diet sweetener in the bunch. I recommend that you completely avoid all artificial sweeteners. They don't have calorie counts because the body doesn't know what to do with them. The body doesn't recognize them because they are foreign substances that have undergone molecular changes. That means *toxicity!* Such substances are not found in nature, and studies continue to prove that they have long-range detrimental effects to our health.

HYPOTHYROID OR SLUGGISH THYROID

Because people with an underactive thyroid tend to have a very low basal metabolic rate. One of the most noticeable symptoms of low thyroid is weight gain and difficulty losing weight. Sometimes an over-active thyroid can mimic an underactive one by causing weight gain, but this is less common. For people with low thyroid who are dieting, their metabolism continues to slow down as calories are reduced. That's why some people with low thyroid can have weight gain even when they severely restrict their calories.

More women than men suffer from a sluggish thyroid, or hypothy-roidism, and many more women than men with thyroid issues have problems with weight gain. Most thyroid problems occur within the gland itself, but it often isn't discovered until other hormonal imbal-ances develop. Often thyroid issues, menopause, and weight gain appear together.

Thyroid problems develop in women more than men for several reasons:

- Often women spend a lot of their lives dieting, usually in a yo-yo pattern of excess eating and strict fasting. This undermines the metabolism and decreases the metabolic rate, a multipart factor impacting the thyroid, especially during perimenopause.
- Women more than men tend to internalize stress, which affects the adrenal and thyroid glands. Over-active adrenal glands produce excess cortisol, which interferes with thyroid hormones and deposits fat around the midsection. In addition, fatigue caused by overstressed adrenals increases cravings for sweets and refined carbohydrates to provide quick energy and feel-good hormones.
- Women's bodies require a delicate balance of hormones such as estrogen and progesterone. These can be upset

when the body is stressed, when it is slightly acidic, or
when it is not getting enough nutritional support. This
results in hormonal imbalances, which act as a trigger
for thyroid problems.

There are a number of symptoms that can be experienced when you
have an underactive thyroid, such as fatigue, depression, weight gain,
cold hands and feet, low body temperature, sensitivity to cold, a feeling
of always being chilled, joint pain, headaches, menstrual disorders,
insomnia, dry skin, puffy eyes, hair loss, brittle nails, constipation,
mental dullness, frequent infections, hoarse voice, ringing in the ears,
dizziness, and low sex drive. If you suspect that you have low thyroid,
you should get tested. However, be aware that you may not test as
hypothyroid, yet you may still have an underactive thyroid gland.
(You can take the Thyroid Health Quiz in my book *The Coconut Diet*.
I have extensive information on thyroid health in chapter 4 of that
book and more than seventy delicious recipes using coconut oil.)

What You Can Do to Nourish Your Thyroid

In order to fix your metabolism, you need to nourish your thyroid
gland and work on your overall health. Here's what you can do.

Consume plenty of iodine-rich foods.

The thyroid uses iodine to make the thyroid hormone. If iodine is
not available in ample amounts in your diet, the thyroid may produce
an insufficient amount of hormone. Agricultural farmland is increasingly deficient in iodine, leading to lower levels of iodine in foods. It's
important to eat iodine-rich foods, including fish, seafood, sea vegetables, eggs, cranberries, spinach, and green bell peppers.

Use Celtic sea salt; avoid iodized sodium chloride (table salt).

Celtic sea salt naturally contains iodine with a full complement of
other minerals that work together. There is no nutrient that occurs
alone in nature. Isolating a nutrient or synthesizing one, as iodine
added to table salt, takes the nutrient out of its natural context. If you
eat too much salt, you can get too much iodine, which causes other
forms of thyroid problems, including iodine-induced hypothyroidism,
autoimmune thyroiditis, and hyperthyroidism. When you consider
all the salt in snack foods, fast food, restaurant food, and packaged
items in addition to what is added to home-cooked food, it's easy to see

how people get far too much iodine and salt. Unprocessed Celtic sea salt contains .000045 percent iodine. If you use 2.5 grams (about 1/2 teaspoon) of Celtic salt daily, you will get around 110 micrograms of iodine. That is more than two-thirds the daily requirement for adults. The remainder of your daily requirement can easily come from kelp and iodine-rich foods.

Take a good multivitamin-mineral supplement.

In addition to iodine, a number of nutrients have been shown to contribute to thyroid health—zinc, selenium, manganese, chromium, B vitamins, vitamin C, vitamin E, and vitamin A. Cod liver oil is a good source of vitamins A and D. (You can get lemon or orange-flavored cod liver oil, which tastes better than plain.) Also, kelp tablets are a good source of iodine, which can support both the thyroid and pituitary glands. Look for Icelandic or Norwegian kelp tablets; the waters in those areas are purer. Selenium is involved in conversion of T4 to T3 hormones. Low selenium levels could lead to low T3 levels. Chromium helps metabolize carbohydrates and fat. It is also important for hormonal activity, especially insulin, and it plays a role in thyroid hormone metabolism. See Appendix A for recommendations on a good multivitamin.

Avoid or limit goitrogens.

A goitrogen is something that blocks iodine absorption by the thyroid gland. The most commonly eaten of these foods are soy and peanuts. Other foods include cruciferous vegetables (broccoli, cauliflower, brussels sprouts, kale, cabbage, bok choy, turnips, and cassava root), pine nuts, and millet. Watch out for soybean oil in salad dressings and snack foods; also textured vegetable protein, which is soy. It's used as filler in a lot of snack foods and energy bars. Use almond, oat, or rice milk instead of soy milk. And avoid soy ice cream, soy cheese, and soy protein powder.

Avoid fluoride.

Fluoride will impede the absorption of iodine. Fluoride is added to city water treatment all across America. Unless you have a special water purification system that takes out fluoride, you will be drinking it. It's added to toothpaste, so you will need to shop for fluoride-free toothpaste. And avoid getting your teeth painted with fluoride at the dental office.

Use virgin coconut oil in food preparation.

Polyunsaturated oils such as soy, corn, safflower, and sunflower oil are damaging to the thyroid gland because they oxidize quickly and become rancid. This happens due to the fact that when oils are stored in our tissues, they are much warmer and more directly exposed to oxygen than they are in the seeds. Therefore, the tendency to oxidize is great. Considerable research has shown that trans fats, present when vegetable oils are processed and heated to higher temperatures, are especially damaging to the thyroid. Because these longer-chain fatty acids are deposited in cells more often as rancid, oxidized fat, the body's ability to convert the thyroid hormone T4 to T3 (which is needed to convert fat to energy) is impaired. When this breakdown occurs, a person can develop symptoms of hypothyroidism.

The opposite effect happens with virgin coconut oil; it does not oxidize and turn rancid easily. It typically has a shelf life of two years. It's a heart-healthy saturated fat that has been used in the tropics for generations with health-enhancing results. It has a unique ability to prevent weight gain and actually helps people lose weight. It helps to raise metabolism because the liver likes to burn it. Since the liver is the primary organ where damage occurs from oxidized and rancid oils that cause cell membrane damage, and where much of the conversion of T4 to T3 hormones take place, replacing the long-chain polyunsaturated oils with the medium-chain fatty acids in coconut oil can, in time, help you rebuild cell membranes and increase enzyme production that will help in promoting conversion of T4 to T3 hormones. Coconut oil got a bad rap for years due to faulty information. For more information on virgin coconut oil, see Appendix A.

Julia Lost Weight With Virgin Coconut Oil

I didn't realize how much hypothyroidism was affecting my life until I started on virgin coconut oil. I suddenly had energy like the Energizer Bunny! I gave up the "white toxins" (wheat flour, refined sugar, potatoes, and other high-glycemic foods). I combined this diet with coconut oil, and it has made a tremendous difference in my hormonal balance, mood, stability, and overall energy. I'm slowly but steadily losing weight. I feel *great*!

—JULIA

Sleep Disorders

Have you noticed that when you don't get enough sleep you have the munchies? Could those nights up late at the computer, watching TV, or restlessly tossing in bed be altering your metabolism?

Studies have shown that people who are sleep deprived eat more food, often choosing the most fattening fare. Dr. Robert Stickgold, associate professor of psychiatry and a neuroscientist specializing in sleep research at Harvard, said, "Up at 2:00 a.m., working on a paper, a steak or pasta is not very attractive. You'll grab the candy bar instead. It probably has to do with the glucose regulation going off. It could be that a good chunk of our epidemic of obesity is actually an epidemic of sleep deprivation."[6]

In the last forty years, the rate of obesity in the United States has nearly tripled to one in three adults. But consider this: over the same period, the U.S. population has subtracted, on average, more than an hour from their nightly slumber and about two hours since 1910, when the average person slept 9 hours a night. According to the National Sleep Foundation, people in the United States typically sleep about 6.8 hours on weeknights (that's about 2 hours less than they did a century ago) and 7.4 hours on weekends.[7]

In a study of the sleep habits of 3,682 individuals, conducted by Columbia University, those who slept less than 4 hours a night were 73 percent more likely to be obese than those who slept 7 to 9 hours nightly. Individuals who slept 6 hours a night were 23 percent more likely to be obese. Other studies have reported that sleeping 6.5 or fewer hours for successive nights can cause potentially harmful metabolic, hormonal, and immune changes that can lead to illnesses and diseases such as cancer, diabetes, obesity, and heart disease.[8]

Research shows that hormones that make you hungry and hormones that control your appetite can be significantly influenced by how much sleep you get. Here's what studies have revealed:

- Five major appetite-influencing hormones can get out of whack when you don't sleep enough, which notably affects how much food you eat.
- Your metabolism can really suffer when you are sleep deprived.

- When you get seven to nine hours sleep per night, your body will better regulate your appetite-suppressing and appetite-stimulating hormones.
- Cravings for high-calorie, carbohydrate-rich foods will diminish when you get refreshing sleep.
- You will be able to manage your blood sugar more effectively when you get sufficient sleep, which helps you manage your appetite. Just one week of sleep deprivation can set off a temporary "diabetic effect," causing you to crave sugar and other fattening foods.
- Extra sleep has its advantages. Research shows that if you increase your sleep by just thirty minutes per night, your chances of losing weight go up exponentially.

Never again feel guilty about sleeping. But what if you want to sleep and can't? There's a lot you can do to correct sleep disorders. Get a copy of my book *Sleep Away the Pounds*, where you will find dozens of remedies to help you correct a host of sleep problems.

You can also check out the amino acid program I discovered a number of years ago when I couldn't sleep. (See Appendix A.) I was actually working on my sleep and weight-loss book when I developed horrible insomnia. I had a urinalysis test done, which showed that some of my major brain neurotransmitters were really out of whack, namely serotonin, dopamine, epinephrine, and norepinephrine. I discovered that when they get that far out of balance, it's very hard to bring them back in balance with diet alone. The right amino acids tailored to my specific needs worked amazingly fast. Within about three weeks, I was sleeping deeply again.

The Amino Acid Program Can Help You Sleep

Amino acids can help balance neurotransmitters that influence sleep. Neurotransmitters are the natural chemicals manufactured in the body from the proteins we consume. They facilitate communication throughout the body and brain. Two neurotransmitters play a very significant role in a good sleep cycle—serotonin and norepinephrine. We need enough serotonin to fully convert to melatonin as well as enough norepinephrine.

When we awake' in the morning, our excitatory or stimulating neurotransmitters, such as norepinephrine, should be high. The excitatory neurotransmitters need to fall all day long for a good sleep cycle to occur at night. Without both serotonin and norepinephrine in balance, restful sleep does not usually occur. If your serotonin is too low or your norepinephrine is too high (or too low), you will have insomnia. When they're balanced, you should get a good night's sleep, which means seven to nine hours of deep, restful sleep for most people.

Serotonin is converted from the amino acid L-tryptophan, which is broken down into 5-hydroxytryptophan (5-HTP) for the creation of serotonin. The body often needs larger amounts of this amino acid than we get from food. Additionally, other cofactors such as B vitamins and enzymes must be present for this to occur. Since L-tryptophan breaks down into 5-HTP at a very low percentage, often 5-HTP is taken as a supplement. Dosages should be based on testing, however. B vitamins are among the necessary nutrients for the creation and transport of L-tryptophan and conversion of 5-HTP into serotonin. They should also be taken as part of a complete brain wellness plan. Omega-3 fatty acids and varied protein consumption are imperative. You may greatly benefit from an amino acid supplement program tailored to your body's specific needs. (See Appendix A for more information.)

Also, be aware that if the liver is congested, you may have a tough time sleeping. I have personally noticed amazing improvements in my quality of sleep after I've completed a liver cleanse. Take heart if sleep has been an issue for you. If you can get to the root of the problem, you can correct a sleep disorder by making the necessary changes.

Sarah Found Cleansing Helped Her Sleep

I had my gallbladder removed twenty years ago, so I have to support my liver and elimination system. If my body gets too toxic, I find myself waking up with a racing mind, even though I'm not under any kind of stress. Good cleansing can help one sleep.

—SARAH

CANDIDIASIS

Candida albicans are usually benign yeasts (or fungi) that naturally inhabit the digestive tract. They are meant to live in harmonious relationship with beneficial intestinal flora. In healthy people, they don't present a problem because they're kept in check by the good gut bacteria.

But when the good bacteria are destroyed by the use of antibiotics or other medications, yeasts flourish. Combine that with many of our twenty-first-century lifestyle habits, such as a diet rich in sugar, refined carbohydrates, alcohol, birth control pills, and stress, and the perfect environment is created that encourages yeast growth that's out of control.

Candidiasis can cause a variety of symptoms, such as cravings for sugar, bread, or alcohol; weight gain; fatigue; vaginitis; immune system dysfunction; depression; digestive disorders; frequent ear and sinus infections; intense itching; chemical sensitivities; canker sores; and ringworm. Some people say they feel "sick all over." If you think you may have a yeast overgrowth, you can take the Candida Quiz in *The Coconut Diet*.

There are a number of things you can do to correct the problem of yeast overgrowth, starting with the list below. Be aware that as yeasts die, your symptoms may worsen for a short time or you may experience some adverse reactions such as headaches or diarrhea. Such reactions are known as the Herxheimer reaction (die-off effect), which is the result of the rapid killing of microorganisms and absorption of large quantities of yeast toxins, cell particles, and antigens. Hang in there. Your health and weight loss will improve if you stick with the program.

- *Follow a candida-control diet.* The Turbo Diet fits the bill because it is low-glycemic and eliminates grains, fruit, alcohol, sugars, and other carbohydrates that quickly turn to sugar, which *Candida albicans* is known to feed on. Even natural sugars like agave syrup, brown rice syrup, or pure maple syrup should be eliminated when cleansing the body of yeasts—and that includes fruit, except for lemons and limes. Sugars are the primary food for yeasts. Milk and dairy products need to be omitted as well because milk lactose promotes overgrowth of yeasts. Also, all mold- and yeast-containing foods such as alcohol, cheese, dried fruit, bread, and peanuts must be completely avoided. Food allergens should also be eliminated.

- *Include virgin coconut oil in your diet.* Research shows that the medium-chain fatty acids in coconut oil kill *Candida albicans.*[9] Caprylic acid is one of the fatty acids found in coconut oil that have been used for fighting *Candida albicans* infections. Besides caprylic acid, two other medium-chain fats (lauric and capric acid) found in coconut oil have been shown to kill yeasts.

  A study at the University of Iceland showed that capric acid causes the fastest and most effective killing of all three strains of *Candida albicans* tested, leaving the cytoplasm disorganized and shrunken because of a disrupted or disintegrated plasma membrane. Lauric acid was the most active at lower concentrations and after a longer incubation time. This study makes the case that all the medium-chain fatty acids in coconut oil work together to kill *Candida albicans.*[10] It is interesting to note that people who eat a lot of coconuts live in areas where yeast and fungi are extremely plentiful, yet they are rarely troubled by yeast infections. Women in the Philippines, who eat their traditional coconut-based diet, rarely, if ever, get yeast infections. Eating coconut oil on a regular basis, as the Filipinos do, helps to keep yeast overgrowth at bay. (For more information on virgin coconut oil, see Appendix A.)

- *Take digestive enzymes.* A major step in treating candidiasis is improving digestive secretions. Gastric hydrochloric acid, pancreatic enzymes, and bile all inhibit the overgrowth of yeasts and prevent its penetration into the surfaces of the small intestine. Decreased secretion of any of these components can lead to a proliferation of *Candida albicans.* Supplementation with hydrochloric acid (betaine HCL), pancreatic enzymes, and nutrients that improve bile flow is crucial in treating chronic candidiasis. The proteases (pancreatic enzymes) are enzymes that break down proteins and are mostly responsible for keeping

the small intestines free of parasites (yeasts, bacteria,
protozoa, and worms). A deficiency in proteases is
also one of the reasons some people experience excessive hair breakage or loss of hair. Supplementation
should include betaine HCL, pancreatic enzymes, and
a lipotropic formula to promote bile flow (the formula
should include choline, methionine, and/or cysteine).
(For a recommendation on enzymes, see Appendix A.)

- *Support the immune system.* A compromised immune
  system leads to yeast overgrowth, and a *Candida albicans* infection promotes damage to the immune system.
  It's a frustrating cycle. You can get tests for immune
  dysfunction, but they are expensive. A practical (and
  free) evaluation is to look at your health history. Have
  you had frequent viral infections including colds and
  flu, outbreaks of cold sores or genital herpes, or pros-
  tatitis in men and vaginal infections in women? These
  are indicative of immune dysfunction. Supplementation with antioxidants, which include vitamins C and
  E, beta-carotene, selenium, and glutathione (found
  in abundance in vegetable juices), along with virgin
  coconut oil, can be very helpful in improving immune
  function.

- *Take probiotics.* Probiotics are strains of beneficial
  intestinal bacteria such as Lactobacillus acidophilus
  and Lactobacillus bifidum, which promote a healthy
  intestinal environment. It's very important that as you
  kill off yeasts, you replace the good bacteria. A good
  probiotic supplement should be part of your wellness
  plan.

Carol Conquered Yeast Problems and Lost Weight

I am a walking testimonial for the benefits of a low-
carbohydrate, high-fat [healthy fats] diet. I had struggled with
Candida albicans and cystitis for years. I used to purchase
Monistat, two or three packages at a time. Now I use lots of
coconut oil for cooking and eat plenty of coconut products
such as fresh coconut, coconut flakes, and coconut milk.
Coconut contains capric, caprylic, and lauric acids—all
proven to kill candida, while leaving healthy intestinal flora

intact. I was taking a long-term, broad-spectrum antibiotic for chronic cystitis for over two years, and now it's been two years since I stopped refilling the prescription with no recurrence! By far the most remarkable transformation occurred when I started using coconut oil and simultaneously eliminated skim milk and all soy products from my diet. And I lost weight.

—CAROL

DIGESTIVE DISORDERS

The major function of the digestive system is to break down and absorb nutrients. When your gastrointestinal system isn't functioning up to par, essential nutrients that are necessary to maintain proper weight and good health may not be absorbed adequately from the foods we eat, even if we are eating a healthy diet. This can lead to nutrient deficiencies, cravings, overeating, weight gain, and poor health.

When you're eating a whole-foods diet and avoiding sugar and other refined carbohydrates, you should not gain weight. However, many people who have switched over to a healthy diet and have even greatly limited their carbohydrate intake still have problems losing weight. You may be one who suffers from poor digestion and experience symptoms like gas, belching, constipation, or a digestive disorder that prevents you from properly breaking down and utilizing your food. You can have the best nutrition on the earth, and it will go to waste unless you are able to digest it well.

When the body suffers from a digestive disorder, it becomes difficult to digest fats. So while it's important to eliminate unhealthy fats from our diet and switch to healthy fats like fish oil, virgin coconut oil, and extra-virgin olive oil, you also need to make sure your digestive system can properly digest the fats you eat. Those with a poorly functioning pancreas have great difficulties in digesting fats. The pancreas produces enzymes that are required for breakdown and absorption of food. For example, lipase, along with bile, functions in the breakdown of fats. Malabsorption (poor absorption) of fat and fat-soluble vitamins occurs when there is a deficiency of lipase.

The digestive system is interrelated, and one poorly functioning aspect of the system usually affects all the others. For example, the liver manufactures bile, which is important in the absorption of fats, oils, and fat-soluble vitamins. When liver function is impaired and there is not enough bile produced, stools can become quite hard and difficult to pass. This affects the health of the colon and increases the absorption of toxins from the stool back into the system. Also, bile serves to keep the small intestine free from microorganisms such as *Candida albicans*, which we looked at previously.

Other digestive disorders include indigestion, irritable bowel syndrome (IBS), gastritis, diverticular disease, dysbiosis (altered bacterial flora), and constipation. More severe digestive disorders are known as inflammatory bowel disease (IBD) and include Crohn's disease and ulcerative colitis, characterized by an inflammatory reaction throughout the bowel. IBD sufferers usually experience bouts of diarrhea, cramping, and weight loss.

Whether or not you have been diagnosed with a digestive disorder, if you have trouble with digestion in any form—burping, bloating, and flatulence to more severe problems such as those mentioned above—chances are that your organs of elimination need detoxifying and your digestive system needs some help. This is especially true as you age. There are a number of steps you can take to improve your digestion.

- *Chew your food very well.* Thoroughly chew each bite of food. Carbohydrate digestion begins in the mouth—chewing food thoroughly allows amylase, the digestive enzyme present in saliva, to digest the carbohydrates.
- *Drink enough water every day; that's about eight glasses.* Not drinking plenty of water is a primary cause of constipation. Constipation promotes an imbalance in bacteria, contributes to inflammation of the intestinal lining, and can even lead to the absorption of larger molecules, a condition known as intestinal permeability. Also, insufficient vitamin C and magnesium can contribute to constipation. Take vitamin C to bowel tolerance (loose stool), and then cut back by about 500 milligrams. This should indicate the amount of vitamin C your body needs. And take magnesium citrate to help improve bowel function. (See Appendix A for more information.)
- *Eat plenty of fiber.* Aim for five to nine servings of vegetables a day. Make some of those vegetables the high-fiber cruciferous veggies like cauliflower, kale,

broccoli, and brussels sprouts. Eat a low-sugar green apple for a snack. Sprinkle ground flaxseeds on your oatmeal or your morning juice or smoothie. Take products with inulin; it's a prebiotic that is good for the colon. (Inulin is a soluble plant fiber that has a slightly sweet taste.)

- *Deal with food sensitivities.* Food sensitivities are behind many digestive disorders. For example, between one-third and two-thirds of IBS patients report having one or more food intolerances, resulting in bloating, gas, and pain. The most common culprits are dairy, grains, corn, and soy.
- *Boost good gut bacteria (probiotics).* Lactobacillus acidophilus and Bifidobacterium bifidum are considered good probiotic bacteria because they can help to maintain intestinal health.
- *Take supplements that restore digestive health.* Enteric-coated peppermint oil can reduce abdominal pain, bloating, and gas. Digestive enzymes will support the body's own digestive enzymes and aid digestion.

Fibromyalgia and Chronic Fatigue Syndrome

Chronic fatigue syndrome (CFS) is a disabling illness that causes extreme exhaustion, muscle pain, sleep disturbances, cognitive difficulties, and hormonal deficiencies and imbalances. Fibromyalgia is a chronic disorder that causes widespread muscle pain, fatigue, sleep disturbances, cognitive difficulties ("Fibro Fog"), stiffness, and headaches. People with these conditions gain weight due to hormonal imbalances, sleep disturbances, and changes in activity levels. Hormonal imbalances, particularly the hypothyroidism found in CFS patients, cause the metabolism to slow down, leading to weight gain. Cortisol, the "stress hormone," is often low during the day but can also start pumping out during the night, causing sleep problems in CFS patients, and this can contribute to weight gain. Cortisol causes weight gain especially around the waist and stomach.

To improve these conditions, you can do the following:

- *Support your adrenal glands.* Most people with fibromyalgia or chronic fatigue syndrome have exhausted adrenal glands. Studies show it's important to normalize blood sugar by eating foods low on the glycemic index; to avoid substances that tax the adrenals, such as caffeine (coffee, black tea, chocolate, soda), alcohol, and sugar; and to include supplements that support the adrenals, such as vitamin C, vitamin B_5, enzymes, and pantothenic acid.

- *Eat a low-glycemic diet.* The Turbo Diet is ideal for fibromyalgia and CFS sufferers since it is low-glycemic and loaded with nutrients that help the body heal. High-carbohydrate foods should be completely avoided and replaced with lean proteins, vegetables, and healthy fats such as avocado, extra-virgin olive oil, and virgin coconut oil.

- *Include foods that are rich in magnesium.* Focus especially on foods that are abundant in magnesium, since low magnesium levels are quite common in CFS and fibromyalgia sufferers. Magnesium is involved in more than three hundred enzymatic reactions in the body, especially those that produce energy. Low magnesium levels equate to low energy. Foods rich in magnesium include legumes, seeds, nuts, and green leafy vegetables, especially beet greens, spinach, Swiss chard, collard greens, and parsley. You may also benefit by including a supplement that combines magnesium and malic acid. (See Appendix A for more information.)

- *Cleanse your body of toxins.* Cleansing is a very important part of correcting these conditions. I know firsthand. Suffering from a devastating case of chronic fatigue syndrome that included chronic pain, I turned my health around completely through juicing, cleansing, and totally changing my diet. You can read my story and my extensive programs for these conditions in my books *The Juice Lady's Guide to Juicing for Health* and *Juicing, Fasting, and Detoxing for Life.* I recommend that if you suffer from either CFS or fibromyalgia, you start a cleansing program as soon as possible.

- *Take two to three tablespoons of virgin coconut oil each day.* The medium-chain triglycerides in coconut oil provide a quick source of energy and stimulate the metabolism. Plus, the fatty acids in coconut oil can kill yeasts and viruses such as Epstein-Barr, herpes, and giardia. With fewer viral organisms taxing the system, the immune system can function more efficiently. I have received reports from fibromyalgia sufferers who have recovered from this terrible disease and are living pain free after starting on the coconut diet and the addition of fresh juice. (See my book *The Coconut Diet.*)

Trudy Dropped 12 Pounds by Juicing and Detoxing

I did a serious detox, with mostly raw foods and juices, along with the help of customized supplements prescribed by my nutritional therapist. Finally, after trying for years, I dropped 12 pounds effortlessly. It made a believer out of me! I don't think I could have lost weight without raw foods and juices.

—TRUDY

OVERLOAD OF CHEMICALS AND TOXICITY

Many people who struggle with being overweight blame themselves for lack of discipline or willpower, but environmental health specialists explain that chemicals in pesticides, plastics, cosmetics, cleaning solvents, and many other commonly used products build up to toxic levels in our bodies and break down our natural defenses and weight-control mechanisms. These foreign substances accumulate in fat cells because that's the safest place for the body to store them. The more chemicals and toxins, the more fat the body holds on to and even manufactures for storage of these damaging substances.

Once toxic material like organophosphates (a compound containing phosphate groups) gets into your body, chances are they will proceed to damage your weight-control systems, making it harder to lose weight in the future. Synthetic chemicals, which have been used to fatten up animals for meat production by reducing their ability to use their own existing fat stores, also contribute to weight gain in humans. Animals fed low doses of organophosphates gain weight on less food. While their use as growth promoters in meat production has been banned after research found them highly toxic, organophosphates remain a common pesticide and are used in the manufacture of gasoline additives, lubricating oil, and rubber. This is just one example of the many toxins in our environment that can disrupt our weight-control systems.

The Turbo Diet is loaded with antioxidants in the juices and whole foods that help detoxify the body and take it from the weight-gain mode to the weight-loss mode.

In addition, there are specific programs designed to detoxify the various organs of elimination in the body. For example, when you detoxify the liver, it will more efficiently metabolize sugars and fats. Getting rid of toxins and boosting your detoxification system is an essential component of long-term weight control and a healthy metabolism. I have an excellent detoxification program in my books *Juicing, Fasting, and Detoxing for Life* and *The Juice Lady's Guide to Juicing for Health* that will lead you step by step in detoxifying your colon, liver, gallbladder, and kidneys.

FOOD SENSITIVITY

Reactions to foods are not always immediate. They can occur many hours after eating with symptoms such as bloating and swelling in the hands, feet, ankles, face, abdomen, chin, and around the eyes. It can also account for bags and dark circles under the eyes. Much of the weight gained is fluid retention caused by inflammation and the release of certain hormones. In addition, there is fermentation of foods, particularly carbohydrates, in the intestines, which can result in a swollen, distended belly due to gas.

Symptoms of food sensitivity can include headache, migraine, indigestion or heartburn, fatigue, depression, joint pain or arthritis, canker sores, chronic respiratory symptoms such as wheezing, sinus congestion or bronchitis, and chronic bowel problems such as diarrhea or constipation.

STRESS

Stress can cause you to gain weight, whereas relaxing can make you thin. Under any physical or psychological stress, the body is designed to protect itself. It stores calories and conserves weight. It pumps hormones like cortisol into your system, which increase blood fats, sugar, and insulin to prepare the body for "fight or flight." It is well known that the excess cortisol released during stressful times causes fat to be deposited in the midsection. Without eating more or exercising less, stress alone will cause weight gain and can lead to diabetes. Active relaxation helps to reduce stress, along with inflammation, and increase fat burning to better control blood sugar.

Chapter 6

Emotional Eating, Binge Eating, and Food Addictions

A S YOU'RE LOST in a dish of the forbidden, drowning your sorrows or cheering your soul, a small voice inside whispers, "What are you doing?" You ignore it and forge ahead with spoonful after spoonful of creamy or crunchy bliss. It's not until later that regret, guilt, and maybe even shame bubble up and you feel completely defeated in your resolve to follow your new healthy juice diet. Truly mad at yourself for just polishing off another helping of the "off limits" stuff, you slip into depression as your self-confidence is peppered with doubt that you can actually pull this off.

Do you ever feel that living with the constant roller coaster of emotional eating, binge eating, and uncontrollable cravings is more than one mere mortal can handle? Well, hold your chin up. There are tools you can use that will help you change your life.

First, you need to understand that you are the answer to your frustration. There's no magic pill to knock out your emotions or obsessions for food. The answers lie within. Changes may come in "bites" as you move forward and let go of old patterns. You may do well for a while and fall off the turbo juice train from time to time. Get up. Keep going. You will reach your goal.

A couple of years ago I worked with a lady on the Turbo Diet plan who was doing just great. She'd lost weight every week and was very encouraged. Then, her cat died. Her grief took the wheel, and she headed down another road. She ate large amounts of high-carb foods, put a bunch of weight back on, and felt so guilty she stopped consulting with me.

This chapter is about how to deal with emotions that derail us, such as sorrow, pain, boredom, sadness, or fear—emotions that so often call for comfort foods. And you can learn to deal with guilt creatively rather than bagging the whole weight-loss plan when you feel like you've messed up big-time.

In the pages that follow, we are going to look at patterns of responding to life's events that have been built around food. It's probably taken years, maybe decades, or even generations of handed-down patterns of eating in your family for these blueprints to establish themselves in your soul. It's going to take some work to reverse them. But you can do it! Just keep in mind, only a very few people have ever been an instant success at changing such patterns. The rest of us have to work at it, make mistakes, set a new resolve, and see the outcome of our bad choices enough times that we know we don't want to experience that anymore.

THE EMOTIONAL TIES THAT BIND

Food is so powerfully connected to feelings that it sometimes seems impossible to consider various foods apart from certain emotions or celebrations. There are many emotions attached to our favorite foods—the joy of celebrations, pain of tragedies, happy moments, sad days, boredom, anxiety, and pleasure. Our favorite foods can be tied to powerful emotions. They connect together a variety of associations that are difficult to separate—memories, emotions, and feelings.

From infancy we have developed deep feelings around food, often buried in the subconscious. When we cried as babies, we were fed; the distress caused by hunger was replaced with a warm, full tummy. As children, food soothed our tears and calmed our fears. As adults, we self-medicate our anxieties, hurts, fears, loneliness, and disappointments. Food is a reliable friend—consistent and dependable. It can be a surrogate for human contact and the bridge by which we form connections.

How many parties or social gatherings have you been to that didn't serve food? Food is the center of celebrations. Think about Thanksgiving, Christmas, Hanukkah, birthdays, the Fourth of July, weddings, dating, and business parties. I'll bet you have a long list of "celebration foods" you enjoy at such times. We all have positive emotions regarding our favorite foods served on special occasions. Most of us also have a list of *comfort foods* that we turn to when we're unhappy, sad, stressed out, or experiencing any number of other emotions. When the going gets tough, we often gravitate to the feel-good foods we remember from our youth—everything from macaroni and cheese to mashed potatoes and gravy, hot bread and butter, chocolate chip cookies (did you eat the dough?), candy, or ice cream.

If your boyfriend dumps you, grilled fish and steamed asparagus probably won't cut it. If you get fired from your job, I'll bet vegetable soup and salad are not what you'll order for lunch. What do you eat when bad things happen? What do you reach for when you're all stressed out? If you're like most of us, you are going to go for foods that are emotionally comforting. And those are usually the fare that's on the "off limits" list.

Many of us have grown up on brand-name products that have little in common with the whole foods from which they were processed. Many times we prefer these foods in times of stress. Even for those of us who have eaten a whole-foods diet for years, there's still, some-where back in the recesses of our soul, fond memories of such things as steaming bowls of canned chicken noodle soup served with a sand-wich made of soft, snowy white bread grilled in margarine and stuffed with melted, orange-colored cheese. Mothers, who were either frazzled by overwork or seduced by the concept of convenience, served high-carb processed foods to us with love, and although they may have been anything but wholesome, in our subconscious mind they're still desir-able and take us back to the comfort of home.

But what is the price of unhealthy comfort foods or simple-plea-sure indulgences? Many of us could say weight gain for one, poor health for another. Unfortunately, all of us who grew up on a diet of brand-name fare and sugar-laden, refined-carb foods have some major rethinking and attitude adjustments to do if we want to successfully adopt a healthy lifestyle that will promote long-term weight management.

We've also grown up with the "bigger is better" mentality in America. It's the "super-size me" idea that's become so popular today in everything from all-you-can-eat buffets to Big Macs and colossal shakes. Have you seen the movie *Super Size Me?* Morgan Spurlock, the film director and subject of the movie, ruins his health in short order eating super-sized, fast-food meals. He cut the project short because of the alarming decline in his blood work and symptoms of poor health. We've come to believe we don't get our money's worth unless it's a

large portion. So when we're dealing with emotional eating or cravings, we not only want our favorite indulgences, but we also want it in
large quantity. Herein lie two challenges—the "off limits" food and the
quantity that we eat.

WHAT TRIGGERS EMOTIONAL EATING?

The stuff that can trigger a flood of emotions is limitless. Maybe it's
a bill you can't pay, a stressful day at work, arguing with a family
member, or getting stood up by a date. When a flood of emotional
energy comes pouring down your psychological pipes, more often
than not the reaction is to run to the fridge for your favorite food and
suppress the whole thing.

At such times you eat food not because you're hungry but because
you're sad, depressed, discouraged, bored, or anxious. That "little
devil" on your shoulder says, "Yep, you're right! It's been a really
crummy day, and you deserve this. Go ahead. Eat a heaping bowl of
ice cream or a large piece of double-chocolate cheesecake. You'll feel a
whole lot better!"

Stress of any kind triggers a drop in serotonin levels, which can
cause cravings for sweets and starches such as cookies, pasta, or bread.
Women are usually more susceptible to stress eating because of fluctuating hormones. PMS can cause women to eat junk food and sweets.
Momentarily, these foods can help improve mood and encourage happy
memories or feelings. (But *momentary* is the key word.) Their lure has
both chemical and emotional triggers. Some foods work on serotonin
levels in the brain, producing a calming effect because they produce
higher levels of serotonin, which is a little like "instant Prozac." Others
work on an emotional level, reminding us of comfort and warmth. But
the effects don't last, and we're often worse off than before we started
eating the junk.

Emotions have roots in the past. You may not be able to consciously
spot the trigger that sends you running to the cupboard or grocery
store, but it's there in your subconscious. You may hear a familiar old
song playing on the radio as you drive home from work. It just happens
that it was *your song* when you and your high school sweetheart were
in love. Then he dropped you for another girl, and you drowned your
sorrows in chocolate chip cookies. All of a sudden you have an insa-
tiable desire to eat chocolate when you hear the song, even though
it's been years since you've thought of that guy. You probably don't

think about him when you hear the song; you just want chocolate! Your mother's admonition of yore, "Don't spoil your dinner!" just flew straight out the window.

Whatever happens in your moments of binge eating, don't be too hard on yourself. Most of the patterns you're working hard to overcome started when you were young. You might not remember where or when they started, but they're there nevertheless. Your earliest memories often revolve around food—calorie-rich, nutrient-light fare. Fear, pain, sorrow, joy, and happiness—almost always these emotions are associated with the really bad stuff: sugar, white flour, and salty snacks.

But don't give up. You can change this pattern. If your brain can grow new dendrites and your liver can rejuvenate itself, you can develop new patterns of eating and behaving.

You Can't Control Everything

When the toilet overflows, the car breaks down, or your computer crashes, you certainly can't know how to fix everything. We think we can manage the universe, but we aren't experts on all fronts. We just can't control it all. When stuff happens, our emotions often spin out of control. That's when we run for our favorite comfort food. For me, it used to be mashed potatoes with a boatload of butter. I even started buying boxes of instant mashed potatoes years ago so that I could make them quickly. (Take heart; there's hope. I haven't bought those in years.) Whatever we eat doesn't solve the problem, as you know, and often makes it worse. Meantime, the problem's still there.

The computer guy probably never wants to eat a bag of chips out of frustration when he's working on a computer problem. But when my computer crashes or my Internet connection goes down, I feel helpless and hopeless. What makes you feel helpless and out of control?

While working on this chapter, my furnace went down. It was cold outside. I didn't want to call the furnace company. It costs sixty-five dollars for them to walk through my front door and tell me that the panels to my furnace don't fit properly, and therefore the little white button is not getting pushed in to turn the furnace on. I face this challenge nearly every time I change the filter in my furnace. I know the panels don't fit right. It's tricky to get them on. Today, it didn't work no matter what I did. But I'm juice fasting today. Just consuming fresh veggie juices and raw soup. I'm not going to break my juice fast simply because I'm frustrated. So I did the one thing that works. It works every single time. I've tried all the clever little suggestions that experts write about that are supposed to help us get through these emotionally upsetting events. None of them have worked for me. But this works.

Prayer. That's right. Prayer. When I can't figure it out, I've learned to pray. So I just simply prayed for a furnace angel to come and help me with a creative idea. Sure enough, I got an idea. Duct tape. (My fix-it angel loves duct tape.) A few strips of duct tape wadded up and stuck in just the right spot of the door panel, and *voilà*! The furnace was humming. A few years ago, I'd have been a wreck, smacking the door panel, freezing, and emotionally tied in a knot. I'd probably have eaten a lot more than a bowl of instant mashed potatoes with butter. But now my problem was solved. I was happy and at peace. I grabbed my big glass of beet, carrot, cucumber, kale, lemon, and ginger juice and sat down to drink my lunch.

Try it! Whether you're sitting at the genius bar waiting for a computer geek to fix your crashed computer and hopefully retrieve all the files you're fearing are permanently lost, or you're sitting on hold waiting for your high-speed Internet server rep to figure out why you can't connect—pray. Pray for the person working on your problem. Pray for creative ideas for the fix-it person. Pray for yourself and your peace of mind. It's amazing what happens. It can change your entire life.

You can't control everything that happens. You can control your reactions. And you can let go and pray.

ADMIT, ACKNOWLEDGE, CONFRONT

You may not have thought a lot about the binge eating you do from time to time. These episodes just happen, right? And life goes on. But life doesn't go on well, and the binges will never change—you'll never change—until you admit that you binge and confront your behavior.

I've written a lot of books, taught numerous classes, and spoken to large groups of people at seminars. People take notes, underline points in my books, and talk a lot about eating the right foods. It's usually emotional eating and binge eating that keep them from the weight they want and the good health they long for.

If you're keeping your binge eating a secret, maybe not even admitting it to yourself, you will stay on that emotional eating roller coaster for a long time. Isn't it time to take a good look at what's going on? How is your mind influencing you? How is your past triggering you? You may be trying to hold that emotional beach ball under water with all your might, but every once in a while the thing just pops up. The volcano of past experiences with the emotions they spawned is buried in your subconscious. These emotions erupt every now and then.

Your story might tear my heart in two. A lot of people who suffer with binge eating, emotional eating, or more serious eating disorders have suffered abuse, deprivation, painful loss, or rejection in their past. Heartbreaking things can happen to us. Life can offer us a rough road to travel. But at some point we have to ask ourselves if we're going to allow what happened in the past to wreck our present and future. While you can't control what happened to you, you can control your response to what happened then and your response to what happens now and in the future.

No matter how many times you have tried and failed to choose a healthy lifestyle, don't lose hope. You can do this. It just takes a willing heart. You have that. That's why you chose this book. You were looking for hope and a plan that would work. Willpower or gutting it out only works so long. Then the whole thing snaps like a broken rubber band. And you're right back to your old behavior. But a willing heart that's open to change and to finding a new way of responding to life—well, that kind of humble approach gets you further than you'd think. A willing heart looks for creative ways and helping angels to get you through the tough moments of life. I promise; you can get through those moments of your life, and you can change.

MY STORY

I experienced a devastating health crisis in my late twenties and had to quit my job when I turned thirty. I had a case of chronic fatigue syndrome that made me so sick I couldn't work. I felt as though I had a never-ending flu. Constantly feverish with swollen glands and perennially lethargic, I was also in constant pain. My body ached as though I'd been bounced around in a washing machine. I moved back to my father's home in Colorado to recover. I juiced and ate a nearly perfect diet for three months. One morning I woke up feeling like someone had given me a new body in the night. Actually, my body had been healing all along; it just manifested at that moment. I looked and felt completely renewed and totally healed. With my juicer in tow and a new lifestyle fully embraced, I returned to Southern California to finish writing my first book. For nearly a year, it was "ten steps forward" with good health and more energy and stamina than I'd ever remembered.

Then, all of a sudden, I took a giant step back.

I was house-sitting in a lovely Southern California neighborhood for vacationing friends of our family and working on my book. It was the Fourth of July.

I woke up around 3:00 a.m., rolled over in bed, and saw a young man crouched in the corner of the bedroom—something every woman I've ever known has dreaded. Instead of running, he leaped off the floor and attacked me, beating me repeatedly with a pipe and yelling, "Now you are dead!" We fought, or I should say I tried to defend myself and grab the pipe. It finally flew out of his hands. He then choked me until I was unconscious. In those last seconds of life I knew I was dying. I felt sad for the people who loved me and how they would feel about this tragic death. Then I felt my spirit leave in a sensation of popping out of my body and floating upward. Suddenly everything was peaceful and still. I sensed I was traveling, at what seemed like the speed of light, through black space. I saw little twinkling lights in the distance.

Then, all of a sudden, I was back in my body, outside the house, clinging to a fence at the end of the dog run. I don't know how I got there. I screamed for help. It was my third scream and took all my strength. I felt it would be my last. Each time I'd screamed, I passed out and then had to pull myself up again. A neighbor heard me that time and sent her husband to help. Within minutes, I was on my way to the hospital.

I suffered serious injuries to my head, neck, back, and right hand, with multiple head wounds and part of my scalp torn from my head. I also incurred numerous cracked teeth that resulted in several root canals and crowns. But my right hand sustained the most severe injuries, with two knuckles crushed to mere bone fragments that had to be held together by three metal pins. Six months after the attack, I still couldn't use it. The cast I wore, with bands holding up my ring finger that was nearly torn from my hand, and various odd-shaped molded parts looked like something from a science-fiction movie. I felt and looked worse than hopeless, with a shaved top of my head, totally red and swollen eyes, a gash on my face, a useless right hand, terrorizing fear, and barely enough energy to get dressed in the morning.

Needless to say, I was an emotional wreck. I couldn't sleep at night—not even a minute. It was torturous. Never mind that I was staying with a cousin and his family. There was no need to worry about safety from a practical point of view, but that made no difference emotionally. I'd lie in bed all night and stare at the ceiling or the bedroom door. I had five lights that I kept on all night. I'd try to read, but my eyes would sting. I could only sleep for a little while during the day.

But the worst was the inner pain in my soul that nearly took my breath away. All the emotional pain of the attack joined up with the pain and trauma of my past for an emotional tsunami. My past had been riddled with loss, trauma, and anxiety. My mother had died of cancer when I was six. I couldn't remember much about her death—the memories seemed blocked. But my cousin said I fainted at her funeral. That told me the impact was huge.

I lived for the next three years with my maternal grandparents and father. But Grandpa John, the love of my life, died when I was nine—the loss was immeasurable. Four years later, my father was involved in a very tragic situation that would take far too long to discuss in this chapter, but I can sum it up by saying it was horrific. He was no longer in my daily life. I felt terrified about my future. My grandmother was eighty-six. I had no idea how many more years she would live. The next year I moved to Oregon to live with an aunt and uncle until I graduated from high school.

As you can probably imagine, wrapped in my soul was a huge amount of anguish and pain with all sorts of triggers for emotional and binge eating. I know firsthand about eating-disorder behavior—binge eating and then not eating anything for a few days. I know what it is to get triggered emotionally and be clueless as to what set off an eating binge. Food is immediate comfort. It's often the first thing we turn to. It was for me. But not wanting to gain a lot of weight, I would then avoid food for a day or two after binge eating.

After the attack, it took every ounce of my will, faith and trust in God, deep spiritual work, alternative medical help, extra vitamins and minerals, vegetable juicing, emotional release, healing prayer, and numerous detox programs to heal physically, mentally, and emotionally. I met a nutritionally minded physician who had healed his own slow-mending broken bones with lots of vitamins and minerals. He gave me vitamin cocktail IVs. Juicing, cleansing, nutritional supplements, a nearly perfect diet, prayer, and physical therapy helped my bones and other injuries heal.

After following this regimen for about nine months, what my hand surgeon said would be impossible became real—a fully restored, fully functional hand. He had told me I'd never use my right hand again and that it wasn't even possible to put in plastic knuckles because of its poor condition. But my knuckles did indeed re-form, and the function of my hand returned. A day came when he told me I was completely healed, and though he admitted he didn't believe in miracles, he said, "You're the closest thing I've seen to one." It *was* a miracle! I had a useful hand again, and my career in writing was not lost.

It was my inner wounds that seemed most severe in the end. Nevertheless, they mended too. I experienced healing from the painful memories and trauma of the attack and the wounds from the past through my own prayers and the prayers of others. I call them the *kitchen angels*. They were the ladies who prayed for me around their kitchen table week after week until I was restored to health. I cried endless buckets of tears that had been pent up in my soul. It all needed release. Forgiveness and letting go came in stages and were an integral part of my total healing. I had to be honest about what I really felt and willing to face the pain and toxic emotions confined inside and then let them go. But, finally, one day after a long journey—I felt free. A time came when I could celebrate the Fourth of July (the anniversary of the attack) without fear.

Today I know more peace and health than I ever thought would be possible. I have experienced what it is to feel whole—complete; not damaged, broken, wounded, or impaired; but truly healed and restored in body, soul, and spirit. And I'm not plagued with emotional eating anymore.

ADDICTED TO AN ADRENALINE RUSH?

Some people look for the excitement of misery, chaos, or crisis. They like pushing the envelope, going to the edge, seeing how far they can take things. Not surprisingly, many of these people grew up in crazy, dysfunctional households with problem parents or siblings or with chaos, trauma, loss, or crisis as a familiar scenario in childhood. They don't know how to function unless things are in turmoil, and they almost panic when things are going well. Have you ever thought that this might be a scenario you experience?

When we think about all the challenging things that have happened in our past, we know we don't want the future to be a repeat. But on a subconscious level, we may be creating repeats over and over again. Psychologists tell us that we can get addicted to the highs and lows of hormone rushes produced by trauma, tragedy, crises, or chaos. Some people are *drama queens*; other people like to stir things up. Some people seem to find themselves in messes over and over again. These are people addicted to chaos or crisis.

Shots of adrenaline and cortisol pump through our bodies at these times and take us back to early days when those hormones pumped through our system like little torpedoes. Though it's not pleasant, we can crave it—become addicted to it. We somehow seek to bring all this familiar emotional and hormonal chaos back. It trashes our body, but we can't see the damage. We just feel the familiar rush. Often, food is tied in with this whole scenario. It may be what we ate during those crisis times that we crave when crisis hits in the present. Indeed, food affects our biochemistry. Many foods and substances can help us achieve those highs and chaotic hormone rushes.

You can overcome food addictions, binge eating, and emotional eating. I've overcome them. Many other people have overcome them. Angela Stokes tells her story in *Raw Emotions* of how her overeating caused her to reach a weight of 300 pounds. She learned how to overcome emotional eating, cravings, and food addictions and lost over 160 pounds. She's taken her life back while actively inspiring others to do the same! She eats a raw food diet and is a strong proponent of a raw foods lifestyle as the path to a healthy life.[1]

Why We Suffer from Emotional Eating

- Emotional pain and a desire to numb the pain
- A desire to stuff emotions
- A desire to hide from emotions
- A perceived need to disconnect from life

MINDFUL EATING

A study done by Duke and Indiana State University found that mindfulness, including specific instructions to slowly savor the flavor of food and be aware of how much food is enough, helped to reduce eating binges from an average of four binges per week to one.[2]

It's rarely easy to make a major change, even when our better sense says this is the best program and the path to fitness. No matter how convinced or motivated we are, there's still a little voice somewhere in our inner depths screaming, "I want sugar-frosted breakfast flakes!" Or whatever was a favorite. And regardless of what foods we choose as a temporary "fix," for our screaming emotions, the positive effects are only momentary. In the end, they set us up for real depression about our weight gain, low energy, or ill health. It's not always easy to make changes, but if we consider that making no change can mean a lifetime of being overweight, unhealthy, and tired, the decision to change becomes compelling.

When an emotional binge strikes, you might want to think about dealing with yourself just as you would a small child who picks up something that could be harmful. Most of us would quickly find something to give the child in exchange for the harmful object so we could then easily take away the thing that could harm him. Start working with yourself in this way. There's an inner child inside of you. Just grabbing the coveted "off limits" food or drink out of your grasp isn't going to work for long. Rebellion will pop up and send you overboard. So rather than trying to force on yourself a strict rule of life, develop your list of exchanges for these moments of cravings. Say you want a cookie. What substitute can you offer yourself that's actually good for you? It might be a dehydrated cracker that has the texture of a cookie. It might be a piece of fruit or something with the fiber inulin, which has a sweet taste. You can say to your inner self, "We can't have that, but we can have this." What can you do when you want ice cream? You can make recipes for frozen desserts that are just fruit you freeze and blend up. I've developed a recipe with veggies—the "Icy, Spicy Tomato Smoothie." It's slushy, spicy, and works for me. You could also freeze coconut water and blend that up. It makes a delicious slush.

Finding Solutions

Ask yourself the following questions when you're tempted to emotionally eat or go on food binges:

- What am I really feeling?
- Can I just be with this feeling?
- If I eat this fattening food or go on a sugar binge, what will it cost me in the long run?
- What's really important to me now?
- What do I want to achieve?
- Is there a better way to take care of myself both emotionally and physically?
- What can I give myself right now that won't cost me my power?
- How can I nurture myself right now without hurting myself?
- If I were a child, how would I really like to be comforted?
- What can I do today that will make me feel good tomorrow?
- How can I reward myself with things that are good for me?

Develop a List of Healthy Substitutes and Rewards

Make a list of healthy food substitutes and keep the foods on hand. What nonfood rewards can you think of that are good for you? Following are a few suggestions:

- Call a friend.
- Take a walk.
- Watch a favorite movie.
- Take a hot bath by candlelight with your favorite music and a cup of herbal tea.
- Work out and work away your worries; exercise can help—it raises endorphins and other "feel-good" hormones.

A Plan of Action

- Get a journal and write about your food cravings; writing about cravings can be helpful. See if you see a pattern as to what triggers them.
- Let your emotions speak rather than suppressing them; write about them.
- Ask your cravings questions. You may be surprised at what you hear. The point is to hear them out and find out what your real need is.
- Food suppresses emotions; allow your feelings and emotions to be heard and understood.
- Think about a trim, healthy person you admire. How do you think that person would handle a food-binge urge?
- Learn to have fun without food.
- Cultivate personal power.
- Increase nurturing life experiences that can help you get beyond junk food and comfort food eating.
- Accept your emotions rather than stuffing them or shutting them down.
- Allow your emotions to come up and let them go.
- Courageously face painful situations and emotions without stuffing them or covering them up.
- Invite nurturing people into your life.
- Cultivate self-loving experiences.
- Practice stress reduction.

Seven Steps You Can Take to Overcome Emotional Eating

1. Get a plan clearly in mind about what you're going to do the next time you're tempted to eat the foods you know aren't on the Turbo Diet.

2. Associate your actions with the outcome of your choices. Be as graphic as you can and try to actually feel what you would experience physically if you ate the things that you shouldn't eat. Or if you experience no adverse physical sensations, think about how this food might impact your

weight. How will you feel when you step on the scale and see you've gained a pound or more?

3. Picture the foods that are detrimental to your weight-loss program with a very negative symbol, such as the words "rat poison" written above them, or any other negative association that will really turn you off.

4. Associate the foods that are part of your weight-loss program with positive thoughts such as, "Mineral water with a slice of lemon is a great party drink! It's better for me than alcohol, and it tastes great!"

5. Develop a list of "right choice" comfort foods that you can turn to when you're emotionally down. Write down a list of acceptable foods for celebrations. Make sure you have some of these foods on hand at all times so you aren't tempted to go out for ice cream or nachos when your emotions are screaming for comfort, when you are anxious and you want to stuff the whole thing, or when you feel like celebrating.

6. The next time you go out to dinner or prepare a special meal at home, and you're tempted to throw caution to the wind and splurge, remember that what you eat will impact your weight and health. Think about how you will feel the next morning when you step on the scale or when you reflect on what you did. You've embarked on a special mission to lose weight and get fit.

7. If you splurge, don't punish yourself. Start over the very next meal with a positive plan to make wise choices in the future. And no matter what, never succumb to the temptation of throwing the whole plan out because you've blown it a time or two. Just pick yourself up and get back in the race!

CREATING THE BODY YOU'VE ALWAYS WANTED

Imagine yourself six months from now with flabby arms and legs, overweight, and discouraged about your appearance. You're fatigued, forgetful, depressed, and catching every "bug" that comes along. How do you feel? Now imagine yourself six months from now with good muscle tone, at or nearing your ideal weight, energetic with plenty of stamina, a positive mental attitude, and vibrant health. How do you feel this time?

The choices you make today will create the fitness and health you will have in the future and the body you will have six months from now. Taking action is key. If you continue in the same old rut, you will get more of the same, and nothing will change. It's time to get going on a new plan of action. Research indicates that people who have active lifestyles appear to have what can be called a "compelling future." This means that having a picture of a positive future can motivate you to do what is necessary to make your desired future a reality.

Here's what you can do right now. Imagine yourself six months to a year from now. We'll call this your "future self." When you see your future self clearly, imagine moving over and physically becoming that person. Now step back and look at your future self again. Ask that future self what he or she wants you to begin doing now to have a more active, healthy lifestyle that can create that future desired self. Whatever your future self says, write it down. Take a look around you. Notice several people who are older than you. Think about them one at a time. Which one is most like the person you'd like to be five, ten, fifteen, and twenty years from now? Which one is closest to living the lifestyle that you would like to have at that age? Write down the activities and health habits that person has developed.

Remember that each day you are creating one of two pictures— your best or your worst self. People who create the best possible future make continual positive decisions for fitness' sake, like juicing vegetables each day and exercising thirty minutes to an hour, three or four times a week. They often use the stairs rather than an elevator and order more salads than sandwiches or pizza. They take more walks. They spend more time in positive pursuits. And they know about deferred gratification. They think about the consequences of daily decisions and how these choices steer them away from or toward their best future self.

Now cut out or draw a picture of your best future self and one of your worst future self. Underneath each picture write down the good or bad habits that would create either person. Put these pictures up where you can look at them every day. Each morning make a decision to choose activities and actions that will correspond with creating your best self. The rewards are immense. It's worth the effort. Every evening look again at the two pictures and evaluate which picture you moved toward that day by your actions.

This isn't an exercise in futility or someone's gimmicky idea that doesn't change a thing. Writing down goals and making collages really do work. It's worked over and over again for me. Years ago I made a collage of my future. I put pictures on an 8 x 11 sheet of paper that included writing books, appearing on television, working with a health institute, and having the money to help people in need. It still hangs in my office. I had only written one book at that time, and none of the other things even seemed remotely possible. To date I've now written seventeen books—this is number seventeen. And everything else has materialized. Two years before I got married, I made a list of all the qualities I wanted in a husband. At the top of the list was priest/psychologist. Guess what! Father John is everything on that list and more. Are you amazed? I am still amazed to this day.

When I met George Foreman in Las Vegas at the Gourmet Product Show in 1995 where they unveiled his new Lean, Mean, Fat-Reducing Grilling Machine that rocked the nation, I was working with Salton, the company that developed that product. I decided then and there that I wanted to work with George to promote the grill as his nutritionist. I got an autographed picture of George and put it up on the bulletin board in my office. Every day as I walked by it, I'd say, "I'm going to work with you on that grilling project." Well, as they say, the rest is history. The company and George accepted my proposal. I appeared in three of the George Foreman Grill infomercials. I appeared on QVC for over eleven years with the grill and was one of the top on-air presenters in housewares on QVC. I also wrote a best-selling grilling cookbook with George.

Now what do you think about writing down your future goals and creating pictures of your best future self?

What kind of body will you need to complete your goals and dreams? What weight should you be at to meet your goals? What level of health do you need to fulfill your destiny?

Your future is in your hands—one choice, maybe one sip of juice or bite of food at a time.

You Have a Purpose

After all that happened to me, including dying and coming back, I knew there was a purpose for my life—a reason I had lived. I could help others find their way to wholeness—body, soul, and spirit. I could help people, maybe you, let go of emotional pain and make healthy choices for life.

There's a purpose for your life. All the pain, trauma, rejection, disappointment, or loss that you've experienced can become the fabric of your stronger soul and the launching pad for a life lived to the fullest. You can reach out to the world with a generous heart and make a difference right where you live and around the world, if that's your goal.

A number of years ago when I was on air on QVC as spokesperson for the George Foreman grills, one of the men in the maintenance department at the hotel where I stayed would drive me in the hotel van to QVC for evening shows. We'd talk about our lives on the way. He may have been a maintenance man by night, but by day he had a special purpose in his neighborhood. Many of the single parents worked long hours. Because he worked the late-night shift at the hotel, he had time to give to neighborhood kids in the afternoon. He and his wife and their children opened their home after school to the kids who had nowhere to go. He'd barbecue for them, play games with them, take them to ball games, and out on Saturday fishing trips in the summer. He gave those kids many happy memories where they would have otherwise been lonely kids maybe getting in trouble after school. Who knows what kinds of problems he saved those kids from experiencing because he was there living his purpose?

Often, as this man related stories of the kids to me, I'd think about purpose. He made me so aware that each of us has a purpose, a place we can make a difference in this world. What's yours? Have you discovered it yet? I'm sure you have more than one purpose.

Why should you work hard to stay at the top of your physical game? Why not succumb to momentary pleasures like grabbing a bag of chips and polishing them off? Or buying a box of Milk Duds for the movie? There's a bigger picture for your life than just getting through a day. You need a healthy, fit, strong body to complete your goals. The temporary "fixes," those little food addictions and cravings that many of us wink at, could be keeping you from the great joy of fulfilling the reason you're here on this earth. There are people waiting for you—*just you*. Nobody else can do what you do.

When you discover and fully embrace your purpose, you will be able to more fully embrace the Turbo Diet way of life and let go of the foods that don't serve you well. If you're clueless as to what your purpose is, pray. That's what I did each time I made a future list or a collage of pictures. In the meantime, get ready physically. You need energy, a fit body, clear mind, and abundant health to complete your goals. You can choose today to live healthy, fit, and strong so you can share your gifts with the world.

Chapter 7

The Turbo Diet Plan

WELCOME TO THE Turbo Diet Menu Plan. You are about to experience weight loss on a healthy mission. The plan includes two glasses of delicious veggie juice every day, plenty of taste satisfaction, and low-glycemic, great-tasting recipes. You're off to a great start! And, like so many Turbo Dieters, you too will be amazed at how you feel.

If you think you will have nothing interesting left to eat on a low-glycemic diet, you will be happily surprised. The Turbo Diet offers delicious foods, juices, and low-glycemic recipes that are part of the fourteen-day meal plan. Actually, the fourteen-day plan is just the launch of a lifetime of healthful eating. It's your "lighthouse" on the troubled sea of bad food choices luring you away from your best and highest goals. If you stray, it's the way you return to pilot home and back to your life-giving choices.

You can choose good carbohydrates from a wide variety of brightly colored vegetables and fruit rich in antioxidants and other important vitamins and minerals that will support your immune system. Lean meat, poultry, fish, and eggs (if you're not vegan), beans, lentils, split peas, seeds, and nuts will give your body the protein it needs.

Healthy fats such as extra virgin olive oil and virgin coconut oil will help you satisfy your hunger faster and more completely. Coconut oil helps boost the body's metabolism. This oil burns quickly, much like kindling in a fireplace. It helps curb cravings, especially for sweets, and keeps hunger at bay.

This is not a diet of deprivation but one of enjoyment. With two to three meals per day, two vegetable juices, and a couple of healthy snacks, you should not feel hungry or deprived. Best of all, you will learn a new style of eating that you can follow for the rest of your life.

The Turbo Diet is not only enjoyable—it's also easy. You are not being asked to measure food or count carbohydrates—just choose from the lists of healthy foods you can eat, and don't eat the foods on the "avoid" list.

Low-glycemic eating will give your body a chance to deal with issues such as insulin resistance brought on by eating too many of the wrong carbohydrates, which are primarily the refined and processed ones. When you no longer experience swings in blood sugar, it should be easier to control cravings for sweets and other high-carbohydrate foods. As a result, you will lose weight faster. Many people on the live foods program choose not to eat animal products. But if you do, make sure you choose the very best.

CHOOSING THE BEST

Before you get to the list of foods you're encouraged to enjoy on the Turbo Diet, let's discuss how to choose the best products among those on the food list. All animal products are not the same; neither are vegetables and fruit, nor anything else on the list for that matter. The "healthy food" issue is where *The Juice Lady's Turbo Juice Diet* differs from many other diet books or weight-loss programs. This is a weight-loss program on a mission. The mission is to help you get healthier and thinner, not just thinner. To that end I'm giving you key information to help you choose wisely when you shop for groceries.

Animal protein

Quality protein is important for your health and weight management. It stimulates the production of glucagon, a hormone that functions opposite insulin. Glucagon stabilizes blood sugar levels and provides brain fuel by signaling the body to release stored energy. When synchronized, insulin and glucagon create a stable hormonal system.

When choosing animal protein, opt for grass-fed (also called pastured) beef, lamb, buffalo, and poultry products whenever possible. You will get healthier meat compared with commercial products—meat that has more "good" fats and fewer unhealthy ones. For example, meat from grass-fed animals has two to four times more omega-3 fatty acids than meat from grain-fed animals. This meat is also richer in antioxidants, including vitamin E, beta-carotene, and vitamin C. Furthermore, pastured meat doesn't have traces of hormones, antibiotics, or other drugs. And it has appreciable amounts of CLA (conjugated linoleic acid), three to five times more than products from animals fed conventional diets.[1] Listen up! Studies have shown CLA to promote weight loss. It's a naturally occurring fatty acid found in animal and dairy fats such as beef, lamb, dairy products, poultry, and eggs. Recent studies have also shown possible health benefits from CLA, such as inhibiting tumor formation, maintaining healthy blood vessels, and normalizing metabolism of glucose.[2]

If you can't find grass-fed meat, do shop for free-range or, at the very least, antibiotic-free beef, dairy, lamb, buffalo, and poultry. The growth hormones injected into factory-farmed animals cause them to gain weight. After all, fattening animals quickly to get them to market means more dollars for vendors. But what does it mean for us? These hormones are not healthful; they are even harmful to us. Natural foods markets such as Whole Foods, Wild Oats, co-ops, and many independent health food markets as well as local farmers have pastured or naturally raised beef, lamb, buffalo, and poultry.

Keep in mind that you can get too much animal protein, which is taxing for the kidneys and can contribute to overacidity in the system. That is why it's best to limit portion sizes between 4 and 6 ounces, with women eating no more than 4 ounces.

Candy for Cows!

Some commercial feedlots are giving stale candy to cattle in an effort to reduce costs of fattening them for market. According to a recent review, milk chocolate and candies such as gummy bears, lemon drops, or gumdrops are a cheap means of fattening cattle. The candy is sometimes given to the animals in their wrappers. According to one article, "The upper feeding limits for candy or candy blends and chocolate are 5 and 2 pounds per cow per day, respectively."[3]

Are you outraged? I am. As long as beef producers are not accountable for the ultimate nutritional value of the meat, they will continue to formulate feedlot diets on a least-cost basis, and American consumers will continue to eat meat that is very inferior in quality—artificially high in fat and low in vitamin E, beta-carotene, omega-3 fatty acids, and CLA.

Red meat

Not all red meat is created equal. In addition to being higher in omega-3 fats and CLA, meat from grass-fed animals is also higher in vitamin E. Studies show the meat from pastured cattle is four times higher in vitamin E than meat from feedlot cattle and, interestingly, almost twice as high as the meat from feedlot cattle given vitamin E supplements.[4] That's beneficial, in that vitamin E is linked with a lower risk of heart disease and cancer. Grass-fed beef is also lower in total fat and particularly the saturated fats linked to heart disease. It's also higher in beta-carotene, the B vitamins thiamine and riboflavin, and the minerals calcium, magnesium, and potassium.

Pasture-Raised Lambs Are Higher In Protein and Lutein and Lower in Fat

A team of scientists from the USDA compared grass-fed lambs with lambs fed grain in a feedlot. They found that lambs grazing on pasture had 14 percent less fat and about 8 percent more protein compared to grain-fed lamb. And check this out! Meat from sheep raised on pasture has shown twice as much lutein (carotene) as meat from grain-fed sheep. Lutein reduces the risk of macular degeneration (a leading cause of blindness) and may also help prevent breast and colon cancer.[5]

Poultry and eggs

Pasture-raised poultry are far healthier than commercial-raised fowl. Pastured poultry are chickens, turkey, ducks, and geese that are raised in bottomless cages or pens on grass where they peck and scratch at the ground and hunt for bugs and seeds along with their grain. Their manure is spread over wide areas of pasture as they are moved. This is better for the birds and the soil.

Sometimes they are mistakenly called free-range chickens. But free-range chickens are still kept in confinement; they are just allowed to "free range" inside their buildings. From egg to adulthood, commercial poultry are housed in confinement with their feet standing in their own manure. They do not get the benefits of fresh air and sunshine or the grass, seeds, and bugs of the pasture.

So what are the health benefits of eating pastured poultry?

- **Clean meat.** Commercial poultry is washed with heavily chlorinated water that leaves a residue on the meat. This is why Russia and the European Union will not buy poultry products from most U.S. processors.[6]
- **Healthier meat.** As far back as the 1930s it has been known that confinement and a grain-only diet significantly reduces the health of the chicken. When put on pasture to eat bugs, grass, and seeds in addition to their grain, and allowed to roam in the fresh air and sunshine, the chickens thrive. This means much healthier muscle meat for the consumer.
- **More healthy fats.** Pastured poultry has more omega-3s than commercial chicken meat and more vitamins E and C and beta-carotene.[7]
- **Hormone, antibiotic, and drug free.** There is growing concern that hormone and drug residues in meat and milk might be harmful to human health and the environment. There may be immunological effects and cancer risks for consumers.[8]
- **Arsenic free.** Commercial poultry are often fed trace amounts of arsenic in their feed to stimulate their appetites. Traces of arsenic can be found in the meat, which we ingest.[9]
- **Meat is tastier.** Ask chefs at high-end restaurants about the difference between pastured and commercial poultry. They will pay more for pastured chicken and other meats because they have a high demand for it. It tastes better than the commercial birds.

Eggs from pastured hens

Eggs contain all eight essential amino acids and are a rich source of essential fatty acids, especially when raised on pasture. They also contain considerably more lecithin (a fat emulsifier) than cholesterol. Additionally, eggs from hens bred outdoors have three to six times more vitamin D than eggs from hens bred in confinement.[10] Pastured hens are exposed to direct sunlight, which is converted to vitamin D and passed on to the eggs. And they are rich in sulfur and glutathione. Pastured poultry also offers more folic acid and vitamin B_{12}. In part, this information comes from a British study published in 1974. At the time, British consumers were concerned about the trend toward factory farming. A detailed study confirmed their suspicions—eggs from free-range hens contained significantly more folic acid and vitamin B_{12}.[11] Look for eggs from chickens that are raised cage-free on pasture, without hormones, and fed an organic diet that includes green grass. When chickens are housed indoors and deprived of greens, their eggs become artificially low in good fats. Eggs from pastured hens can contain as much as ten times more omega-3s than eggs from factory hens.

For pastured poultry, look to co-ops and natural food markets; also seek out local producers, farmers, and homesteaders who pasture their poultry or let them roam free.

Lab Tests on Eggs from Pastured Chickens

Mother Earth News collected samples from fourteen pastured chicken flocks across the country and had them tested at an accredited laboratory. The results were compared to official USDA data for commercial eggs. Results showed the pastured eggs contained an astounding:

- One-third less cholesterol than commercial eggs
- One-fourth less saturated fat
- Two-thirds more vitamin A
- Two times more omega-3 fatty acids
- Seven times more beta-carotene[12]

Fish

When it comes to fish, buy wild-caught as often as possible. Farm-raised fish get by almost as poorly as factory farm animals. They are often given antibiotics, raised penned in crowded pools, and not fed their customary diet. Hence, they do not have the essential fatty acids that wild-caught fish offer and that are so important for our health.

When it comes to animal fat, fish is a good source of the healthy omega-3 fatty acids, especially cold-water fish such as salmon, mackerel, and trout, if they're wild caught. Also, the smaller the fish, the less mercury and other heavy metals that will be stored in the flesh.

Vegetable juice, tea, and other beverages

Freshly made vegetable juice is the core of the Turbo Diet. You will drink two glasses of delicious veggie juice each day to facilitate effective weight loss. It's best to drink one glass of veggie juice in the morning and one before dinner. The morning juice helps energize your body and gives you super nutrients to last all morning; the evening juice helps curb your appetite and gives you energy to make a healthy dinner. If this schedule isn't possible, then drink the juices whenever you can. You can make them the night before and take juice to work in a stainless steel water bottle or thermos. You can store juice in a covered container in the refrigerator up to twenty-four hours. Choose organic produce for the healthiest juice. When you absolutely can't juice, you can head to a juice bar. If that's not possible, check out the cooler section of your local grocer for vegetable juices or choose low-sodium V-8 juice.

Freshly made raw, vegetable juices are alkaline producing. (I don't recommend fruit juice because of the sugar. But especially avoid processed fruit juices; they become more acidic when processed and especially when sweetened.) In addition to being an effective part of a weight-loss regimen, vegetable juicing promotes health in a variety of other ways. The concentration of vitamins, minerals, and enzymes that juicing provides gives the body extra stamina as well as a boost to the immune system. This can be of great value when you're trying to lose weight.

Green tea is especially helpful for weight loss. Rich in antioxidants and the phytonutrients catechins and other polyphenols that protect you against inflammation, cancer, and other ailments—green tea is also *thermogenic*. *Thermogenesis* is the production of heat, meaning it revs up your metabolism. Most of the thermogenic action in green tea is due to epigallocatechin gallate (EGCG), which is a potent polyphenol. EGCG also appears to increase the effectiveness of weight-loss supplements such as 5-HTP and tyrosine. For these reasons it's a great idea to make green tea part of your daily meal plan. Strive for at least one cup of healthy tea per day. A cup of green tea has about one-third of the caffeine found in a cup of coffee. Avoid green tea if you are sensitive to caffeine, have low adrenal function, or are hypoglycemic. White tea has less caffeine and may be better tolerated. Herbal teas are also a great choice. When choosing green, white, and herbal tea, look for organically grown. And unbleached tea bags are better choices over bleached.

For bubbly water, choose sparkling mineral water that is naturally carbonated over commercially gassed varieties, such as S. Pellegrino and Apollinaris. If you suffer from IBS, it's advisable to completely eliminate carbonated drinks from your diet in order to allow the GI lining to heal.

Be sure to drink plenty of water. It's recommended that you drink at least eight 8-ounce glasses of water per day to facilitate your weight loss. Purified water is best. Be aware of plastic toxins that are leached into the water from the plastic bottles. Take water with you in stainless steel water bottles. A good water purifier is a great investment.

Completely avoid soft drinks; they are like drinking liquid candy. They're loaded with sugar. Studies have connected them with weight gain and numerous health problems. They're also very acidic. Also, watch out for sweetened teas, energy drinks, sports drinks, and vitamin-infused water. And always avoid diet sodas due to their detrimental health effects and the fact that studies show artificial sweeteners actually cause people to gain weight.[13]

Fats and oils

The best oils are virgin coconut oil and extra-virgin olive oil—virgin coconut oil for cooking and extra-virgin olive oil for cold foods and salad dressing. Coconut oil is much more durable than other oils and doesn't oxidize as easily when heated. Completely avoid polyunsaturated oils such as corn, safflower, sunflower, canola, and soy. All these oils oxidize when heated, which causes inflammation in the body. Inflammation produces insulin resistance. Insulin resistance produces weight gain. Weight gain generates inflammatory cytokines leading to more insulin resistance and more weight gain.

It's recommended that you consume 2–3 tablespoons of virgin coconut oil a day for accelerated weight loss. Coconut oil helps you lose weight. It's thermogenic. The liver likes to burn it, which means it raises the metabolism. It acts like kindling on a fire rather than a big old log. On the other hand, the body likes to store other fats.

Be choosy when it comes to your coconut oil. Many commercial-grade coconut oils are made from *copra*, which means the dried kernel (meat) of the coconut. If standard copra is used as a starting material, the unrefined coconut oil extracted from copra is not suitable for human consumption and must be refined. This is because most copra is dried under the sun in the open air in very unsanitary conditions where it's exposed to insects and molds. Though producers may start with organic coconuts and even label their coconut oil organic, the end product of some brands is refined, bleached, and deodorized oil. High heat and chemical solvents are usually used in this process.

If you use virgin coconut oil made by hand the old-fashioned way, you will immediately notice the difference in taste, smell, and texture from oil made with standard copra. The traditionally made oil, which is known as virgin coconut oil, is far superior in every way. You will pay more for this oil, but it's well worth it.

Olive oil is called *virgin* if it is extracted by means of pressure from millstones. Virgin olive oil is not treated with heat or chemicals. Batches of olives are pressed more than once to produce numerous batches of oil. The first pressing known as *extra virgin* is the most flavorful and has the least acidity. The first cold pressing also has the highest amount of fatty acids and polyphenols (antioxidants). Olive oils from the Mediterranean, and particularly Spain, are the highest in antioxidants. The very best choice is extra-virgin, cold-pressed olive oil that is organically grown in the Mediterranean.

If you do use a little butter, look for raw, cultured butter from dairy cows that have been raised on pasture. It's richer in vitamin A and CLA when it comes from grass-fed cows. Use butter more sparingly than the oils. Completely avoid margarine; it's made from oils that oxidize in the process, may contain trans fats, and is a very unhealthy choice.

Fruit, vegetables, and legumes

In order to choose the very best fruit, vegetables, and legumes, opt for organic produce as often as possible to avoid toxic pesticides and to enjoy increased nutrition. In 1995 the USDA tested more than ten thousand fruit and vegetable samples, with two out of three samples containing pesticide residue.[14]

Plants absorb nutrients from the soil; they also take up pesticides. Healthy soil is rich in minerals and alive with microorganisms. Pesticides kill these much-needed microorganisms. And chemical fertilizers do not replenish the soil in any manner close to traditional composting and other natural practices that nourish soil.

The quality of protein in grains and vegetables is related to the amount of nitrogen in the soil. When there is a lot of nitrogen in the soil, plants increase protein production and decrease carbohydrate synthesis. When the metabolic protein requirements are satisfied, the remaining protein produced is stored in the form of protein that contains fewer essential amino acids. The result of high levels of nitrogen, as found in conventional chemical fertilizers, is an increase in the amount of protein but a reduction in its quality. Organically managed soils release nitrogen in smaller amounts over a longer time than conventional fertilizers. As a result, the quality of protein from organic crops is better in terms of human nutrition.

While organic foods are always the best option in terms of avoiding pesticides, studies also show they are higher in nutrient content. In a 2001 study published in the *Journal of Complementary and Alternative Medicine,* organic produce, on average, contained 27 percent more vitamin C, 21 percent more iron, and 29 percent more magnesium than conventional produce, and all twenty-one minerals compared in the study were higher in the organic produce.[15]

The more nutrient-rich foods you eat, the more your body will be satisfied and cravings will diminish. In this respect, organic produce is helpful for weight loss. But the most important reason to choose organically grown food is for your health.

- **Fruit.** One of the best fruits you can choose is avocado. (Yes, avocado is a fruit.) It's an excellent source of essential fatty acids and glutathione (a powerful anti-oxidant), and it offers some protein. It contains more potassium than bananas (which are off the list until you reach your weight-loss goals), making it an excellent choice for heart disorders. Choose the lowest-glycemic fruit such as cantaloupe, cherries, grapefruit, apples (especially green), and berries. Look for unsweetened cranberry concentrate or pure cranberry juice and lemon and lime juice to flavor water and juices.
- **Vegetables.** Most vegetables are on the list of foods you can enjoy. Eat lots of the brightly colored veggies because they're packed with satisfying nutrients. Eat plenty of salads, sprouts, vegetable sticks, and steamed vegetables, along with veggies incorporated into raw-food dishes. Avoid baked vegetables as much as possible since the sugar content is highest when they're baked. Limit high-starch vegetables such as potatoes, yams, and acorn squash to no more than three times per week; avoid white potatoes until you reach your weight-loss goal. If you are dining out or it's a special occasion

and you just can't resist a potato, the best choice is red
potatoes (less carbs). If you do succumb to a baked
potato, which is very high in carbs, eat it with a fat like
butter. This will help to slow down the rate at which
sugar enters your bloodstream.

- **Legumes (beans, lentils, split peas).** The outer casing
  of legumes (fiber) does slow down the rate at which
  sugar enters your bloodstream, but it's still recommended that you limit beans, lentils, and split peas to
  no more than about three 1-cup servings per week for
  the first three weeks.

Salt

Choose only Celtic sea salt or gray salt. Whole sea salt has a mineral
profile that is similar to our blood. Regular table salt is highly refined
sodium chloride that usually contains additives to make it pour easily.
When salt is processed, minerals are removed. Then, anticaking chemicals such as potassium oxide or aluminum calcium silicate, iodine,
and dextrose (sugar) are added to make table salt. Eat salt sparingly. It
causes the body to retain water and causes us to fluff up.

Spice Up Your Meals!

Incorporate plenty of spices into your recipes, like black
pepper, cayenne, ginger, allspice, cardamom, cinnamon,
coriander, and turmeric. All of these spices have been
shown to induce thermogenesis, which means they help
you metabolize fat. Cumin, chili powder, garlic powder, and
onion powder are other spices you can use to support the fat-
burning process. Allspice, basil, cumin, fennel, peppermint,
sage, thyme, and turmeric improve brain function. You can
add them often to your recipes. Not only will you assist your
body in burning fat, but you will also help your brain function
more efficiently and help prevent diseases like cancer.

Spices give your taste buds lots of satisfaction. Often we
keep eating because our taste buds are yearning for more
flavor. Spices also send a signal to the brain that we are
well nourished and fulfilled. Since biblical times, spices have
been important in the preparation and preservation of food
They were traded like gold in ancient times because people
valued the pleasure they added to their meals. Merchants
traveled the spice routes of the Middle East with their valuable
commerce, selling the flavors that satisfied their customers.
In our culture, we eat more bland food, often flavored with
just fat, salt, or sugar. But our bored, starved taste buds long

for more. So we keep eating, hoping for satisfaction. Spicing up your meals creates a taste adventure that could help you control your appetite!

How to Sweeten Naturally

To sweeten naturally, try using natural fruit juice such as apple, orange, blueberry, or pear. You can add small bits of dried apple, pineapple, shredded coconut, or currants (smaller than raisins). Sprinkle with cinnamon, nutmeg, or cloves. Add a drop or two of stevia (a drop goes a long way).

THE TURBO DIET HEALTHY FOODS LIST
(FOODS TO CHOOSE AND FOODS TO AVOID)

VEGETABLES AND LEGUMES

Choose *Prepare raw, lightly steamed, or grilled*	Limit *until you reach your weight-loss goal*	Avoid
Artichokes	Acorn squash	Baked and refried beans
Asparagus	Beans, all	Breaded, fried, deep-fried, or sautéed vegetables
Bamboo shoots	Corn	Olives, packed in oil
Beets and beet greens	Lentils	Potatoes, white
Beans (green and yellow wax)	Sweet potatoes	Sweet pickles
Bok choy	Peas (split, black-eyed)	
Broccoflower	Potatoes (purple, red)	
Broccoli	Yams	
Broccoli rabe		
Broccolini		
Brussels sprouts		
Cabbage (Chinese, green, red, savoy)		

VEGETABLES AND LEGUMES

Choose *Prepare raw, lightly steamed, or grilled*	Limit *until you reach your weight-loss goal*	Avoid
Carrots		
Cassava		
Cauliflower		
Celery		
Celeriac		
Chard		
Chayote		
Collards		
Cucumber		
Dandelion greens		
Eggplant		
Endive		
Fennel		
Jicama		
Kale		
Kohlrabi		
Lettuce, all varieties		
Mushrooms, all varieties		
Mustard greens		
Okra		
Onions		
Parsley		
Pea pods		
Peppers (red, green, yellow, purple)		
Radicchio		
Radishes, all varieties		
Rutabaga		
Sauerkraut		
Scallions		
Sorrel		
Soybeans (edamame, organic only)		
Spinach		
Sprouts		
Squash (Hubbard, spaghetti, summer/yellow, zucchini)		
Tomatillo		

VEGETABLES AND LEGUMES

Choose *Prepare raw, lightly steamed, or grilled*	Limit *until you reach your weight-loss goal*	Avoid
Tomato (though considered a vegetable, is actually a fruit, classified a berry), all varieties		
Taro		
Turnips		
Water chestnuts		
Watercress		

FRUITS

Choose	Avoid
Apple	Banana
Apricot	Candied fruit
Blackberries	Canned fruit
Blueberries	Dates
Cantaloupe	Dried fruit
Cherries	Grapes, all types
Coconut	Mango
Grapefruit	Persimmons
Honeydew	Plantain
Kiwi	Raisins
Melon	Watermelon
Nectarine	
Orange	
Papaya	
Peach	
Pear	
Pineapple	
Plum	
Raspberries	
Strawberries	
Tangelo	
Tangerine	

PROTEIN

Choose		Avoid
Vegan	Animal *Prepare baked, broiled, grilled, or steamed*	Animal *Completely avoid all breaded, fried, and deep-fried foods*
Beans	Beef: lean cuts are best, such as flank, ground beef (less than 10% fat), New York strip, sirloin, tenderloin, top round	Beef, all fatty cuts more toxins are stored in fat than muscle)
Lentils	Bison (buffalo)	Bacon
Organic tofu (in small amounts)	Calamari	Buffalo wings
Nuts	Chicken (skinless breast and thighs are best)	Canadian bacon
Split peas	Clams	Fish sticks
	Cornish game hen	Fried chicken
	Crab	Ground beef (greater than 10% fat)
	Eggs	Hot dogs (beef, chicken, pork, turkey)
	Elk	Jerky, beef and turkey
	Fresh wild-caught fish, all types	Liver
	Lamb	Liverwurst
	Mussels	Pork (especially bacon and honey-baked ham)
	Oysters	Processed poultry products
	Turkey (skinless is best)	Salami
	Turkey bacon (limit two slices)	Sausage
		Seafood (canned in oil)
		Turkey bacon
		Turkey sausage

DAIRY AND DAIRY ALTERNATIVES

Choose antibiotic-free, preferably organic	Avoid
Alternative milk (almond, hemp, oat, rice)	Cottage cheese
Cheese (best choices are almond, feta, goat, rice)	Cream, half-and-half
	Cream cheese, all types
	Frozen yogurt
	Ice cream, all types
	Milk
	Most cheese (except for Choose list)
	Sour cream
	Yogurt

BEVERAGES

Choose	Avoid
Green tea	Alcohol (beer, wine, mixed drinks)
Herbal tea	Beverages with artificial flavors or sweeteners
Mineral water with lemon, lime, or unsweetened cranberry concentrate for flavor	Beverages with sugar, high-fructose corn syrup, or other sweeteners
Vegetable juices	Chocolate drinks, cocoa
White tea	Coffee
	Diet sodas
	Flavored water, sweetened
	Fruit juices
	Sodas
	Soy milk (a goitrogen)
	Sports drinks

GRAINS, BREADS, AND CEREALS

Choose	Avoid
100% sprouted whole grain	Bagels, all types
Barley	Biscuits
Brown rice	Bread (except for Choose list)
Buckwheat groats	Bread crumbs
Muesli (no sugar or dried fruit added)	Bread sticks
Oat bran	Chips, all types

GRAINS, BREADS, AND CEREALS

Choose	Avoid
Oat bran bread	Corn bread
Oatmeal, steel cut	Crackers, all types
Rice bran	Croissants
Rye, whole	English muffins
Unsweetened bran cereals	Granola, all types, and other cereals (except for Choose list)
Wild rice (cereal grass)	Melba toast
	Muffins, all types
	Pancakes
	Pasta and noodles, including ramen style
	Pita bread
	Popcorn (until you reach your goal weight)
	Popcorn cakes
	Pretzels
	Rice (white, fried, Spanish)
	Rice cakes
	Rolls (dinner rolls; hamburger, hot dog buns)
	Soups (cream-based, noodle, pasta types)
	Taco shells
	Tortillas
	Waffles

FATS AND OILS

Choose	Avoid
Coconut oil (virgin, organic)	Canola oil
Olive oil (extra virgin, organic)	Corn oil
	Peanut oil
	Safflower oil
	Sesame oil
	Soybean oil
	Sunflower oil

NUTS, NUT BUTTERS, SEEDS, AND SEED BUTTERS

Item	Amount
Almond butter	1 tsp.
Almonds	Fewer than 24
Brazil nuts	Fewer than 6
Cashew butter	1 tsp.
Cashews	Fewer than 6
Hazelnut butter	1 tsp.
Hazelnuts	Fewer than 12
Macadamia nut butter	1 tsp.
Macadamia nuts	Fewer than 12
Pecan halves	Fewer than 24
Pine nuts	Fewer than 24
Pistachios	Fewer than 24
Pumpkin seeds	Fewer than 2 Tbsp.
Sesame seeds	Fewer than 2 Tbsp.
Sunflower seeds	Fewer than 2 Tbsp.
Tahini (sesame seed butter)	1 tsp.
Walnut halves	Fewer than 12

It is not recommended that you eat more than the suggested servings per day unless you are following the all-raw diet plan. If you combine nuts and seeds, keep the serving size in mind because nuts and seeds have carbohydrates, as well as protein and fat. Peanuts are not recommended since they are a goitrogen, meaning they have substances that block iodine absorption. Only a small amount occasionally should be eaten.

Note: You may have two dehydrated seed crackers per day in place of nuts or seeds; most of them also have vegetable fiber added. Seed crackers are dehydrated and considered a raw food; most are made without any grains. Some health food stores carry them. You can also make them in a dehydrator. See pages 198–199 for recipes for dehydrated crackers. Some of the raw recipes have nuts in them. If you choose one of these recipes, then choose a cracker without nuts and avoid nuts as a snack that day.

SUGAR, SUGAR SUBSTITUTES, AND SWEET TREATS

Choose	Avoid
Fresh fruit	Agave syrup
Frozen coconut water	Artificial sweeteners, all
Seeds (sunflower, pumpkin)	Brown rice syrup
	Brown sugar
	Brownies
	Cakes
	Candy
	Candy bars
	Cane juice
	Chocolate
	Cookies
	Corn syrup
	Dextrin
	Doughnuts
	Energy bars
	Frozen treats
	Frozen yogurt
	Gelatin
	High-fructose corn syrup
	Honey
	Ice cream
	Maple syrup, pure
	Molasses

Most of the sugar we eat is disguised in sodas and other drinks, desserts, boxed cereals, energy bars, packaged foods, snacks, and yogurt. Much of it is high-fructose corn syrup, which is used to sweeten everything from crackers, tomato sauces, ketchup, sodas, processed meats, and even some health food products. It's used primarily because it's cheap. But many health professionals attribute it to the increase in obesity, metabolic syndrome, diabetes, certain cancers, and heart disease. The more you avoid sugar, the less you will crave it. And you'll lose weight!

Check out the Web site www.sugarshock .com. You will learn about journalist Connie Bennett's journey to a changed life. She suffered from dozens of debilitating symptoms for years. Finally a doctor connected her condition to overeating processed carbohydrates and sweets, which included her favorites—red licorice, chocolate, and hard candy.

For the sake of your health, not just your weight, completely avoid all artificial sweeteners, including Splenda and NutraSweet. These sweeteners cause a host of health problems. And if you think they're helping you lose weight, take a look at the research. People on sugar substitutes actually gain more weight than those using sugar.[16] And using sugar is a very bad choice for your weight as well as your health.

Check out the movie *Sweet Misery* for an eye-opening report on aspartame (NutraSweet). Dr. Woodrow C. Monte says, "Methanol [one of the breakdown products of aspartame]...is considered a toxicant. The ingestion of two teaspoons is considered lethal in humans."[17] Long-term use of aspartame may cause many neurological disorders and other illnesses, including brain cancer, Lou Gehrig's disease, Graves disease, chronic fatigue syndrome, multiple sclerosis, and epilepsy.[18]

SUGAR, SUGAR SUBSTITUTES, AND SWEET TREATS

Choose	Avoid
	Mousse
	Pastries
	Pies
	Pudding
	Sorbet
	Succanot
	Sucrose (white sugar)
	Sugar alcohols (i.e., sorbitol, manitol)
	Tofu frozen dessert
	Whipped topping
	Xylitol

James Turner, chairman of Citizens for Health, has declared that the FDA should review their approval of Splenda based on a study of sucralose that reveals shocking new information about the potential harmful effects of this artificial sweetener on humans. Hundreds of consumers have complained about side effects from using Splenda. The study, published in the *Journal of Toxicology and Environmental Health*, confirms that the chemicals in the little yellow packages should carry a big red warning label, said Turner.[19] It was found that Splenda reduces the amount of good bacteria in the intestines by 50 percent, increases the pH level in the intestines, contributes to increases in body weight, and affects the P-glycoprotein (P-gp) in the body in such a way that crucial health-related drugs could be rejected.[20] The study is clear–Splenda can cause you to gain weight!

CONDIMENTS

Choose	Avoid
Extra-virgin olive oil	Bacon bits
Garlic	Commercial salad dressings made with polyunsaturated oils
Herbs	Croutons
Horseradish	Fruit jams, jellies, marmalades, preserves
Hummus	Fruit sauces
Lemon juice	Ketchup
Lime juice	Lard
Mayonnaise	Margarine
Mustard	Peanut butter
Olives, packed in water	Pickles (except dill)
Onions	Sandwich spreads
Pickles, dill	Shortening, vegetable
Salsa	Sour cream
Sauerkraut	Sweet pickle relish
Shallots	Syrup, all types
Spaghetti sauce, sugar free	
Spices	

CONDIMENTS

Choose	Avoid
Tahini	
Virgin coconut oil	

Guidelines for Servings Per Day

- Protein–animal or vegan: 4–6 ounces per meal
- Eggs–no more than one per day
- Legumes–three 1-cup servings per week
- Grains–two to three 1-cup servings per week
- Nuts, seeds, nut butters–twenty-four small seeds; twelve medium size such as almonds; six large nuts such as macadamia; 1 teaspoon nut butter
- Fruit–one or two servings per day
- Vegetables–unlimited
- Sweetener–small amount of stevia

Don't Forget Your Vitamins

When you're cutting back on food in general, and certain foods such as fruit and grains in particular, it's important to fill in the gaps with a good multivitamin capsule. Be aware that not all supplements are high quality. You will pay a little more for a natural high-quality supplement, but it's worth it.

Happy Mood

When we're happy, we usually eat less. A 1990 study found that selenium promoted a sunnier disposition! In this study, volunteers were given either 100 micrograms of selenium or a sugar pill. Those who were given the selenium noticed an improved mood in just two weeks.[21]

Supplements to Boost Weight Loss

Enzyme supplements

Digestive enzymes can play a big part in weight control. A lack of enzymes is a hidden factor in obesity. Enzymes are essential for supporting healthy weight loss. Lipase is an enzyme that is abundant in raw foods, and since very few of us have a diet rich in raw foods, we lack sufficient amounts to digest normal amounts of fat in our diets. When we eat diets rich in fat but low in enzyme-rich raw food, our bodies can't burn this extra fat as efficiently or turn it into energy. When we have enough lipase, our bodies are able to break down and utilize the fat. Without this vital enzyme, fat accumulates and is stored in arteries, organs, capillaries, and, of course, fat cells. You will see it pack onto your hips, buttocks, stomach, and thighs.

NASCAR Driver Lost 60 Pounds

At the height of my unhealthy living, I weighed 217 pounds. Today I weigh around 160 pounds. Surprisingly, it only took a few months to lose nearly 40 of those pounds. It was totally a result of focusing on eating healthy foods and drinking vegetable juices. I never counted calories, measured my food for quantity, or attempted to keep myself from consuming a certain amount of food.

What started my weight-loss journey was actually a health crisis. At the age of twenty-nine, I was diagnosed with metastasized melanoma and was given a 5 percent chance of living past my thirties. I was devastated. My wife and I wanted to start a family. I had just begun racing on the NASCAR circuit. There was a lot I had to live for. Therefore, I decided I would educate myself on what types of food would bring my body life, wellness, and healing. I ate as much of those foods as I could get my hands on. I juiced the produce, and I ate a lot of it raw as well. I have now enjoyed thousands of salads, and I look forward to each one. I never felt like I was limited to eating "just this" or "just that." Instead, I focused on what I could eat and where I could enjoy freedom in my nourishment.

Within three months, I had lost 40 pounds. But the best news was that after surgery and my dietary changes, my doctor said that all looked good and that "whatever I was doing, I should keep it up." About a year later there was no sign of recurring melanoma. I had also lost another 20 pounds. Best of all, I felt great. I had found a way of life I wanted to stick with for the rest of my life.

—Jerrod Sessler
Author of Five Percent Chance

Protease is a vital enzyme for breaking down proteins and eliminating toxins. If your body is storing toxins, it becomes more difficult to burn fat—fat cells are where your body stores excess toxins. When you do burn fat, toxins are released back into your system, which can cause water retention and bloating. So a diet rich in protease, or enzyme supplementation, will help to eliminate toxins, which is why these two enzymes are so important when you are losing weight.

Amylase is an enzyme that breaks starch down into sugar. Amylase is present in human saliva—the mouth is where the chemical process of digestion begins. Amylase assists in the digestion of starches and carbohydrates and, when combined with the other enzymes, supports overall digestion. It also serves as a glucose balancer. This is one reason it's so important to chew your food very well.

Calcium

One study found that a diet consisting mainly of high-calcium foods resulted in an average weight loss of 24.6 pounds in sixteen weeks.[22] This is greater than the average weight loss in one year in trials using weight-loss drugs. According to the *Journal of the American College of Nutrition*, fifty-four young women participated in a two-year study; those with the highest intakes of calcium lost the most weight and body fat on weight-control programs, regardless of exercise level.[23] Other peer-reviewed trials continue to indicate that high-calcium diets are associated with lower body weight. In another study, researchers estimated that only 1,000 milligrams of additional calcium intake daily resulted in a 17.6-pound difference in body weight.[24] (See Appendix A for calcium recommendations.)

Vitamin D

A University of Minnesota study has found that higher levels of vitamin D on a low-calorie diet may help people lose more weight, especially around the abdomen. The study found that subjects lost a quarter to a half pound more fat when their vitamin D level was increased.[25] (See Appendix A for vitamin D recommendations.)

5-hydroxytryptophan (5-HTP)

5-HTP is the immediate precursor to serotonin and has been studied in the treatment of obesity. One study concluded that 5-HTP reduced the total number of daily calories without a conscious effort to lose weight by any of the female participants. Average weight loss in this particular study was 3 pounds over the course of five weeks.[26] A second study involved a six-week period without dietary restriction and the second six weeks with the addition of a 1,200-calorie diet. There was a marked increase in weight loss of participants taking the supplement versus those given a placebo. The average weight loss was 10.3 pounds for the supplement group and 2.28 pounds for the placebo group. The conclusion was that 5-HTP's action on the satiety center of the brain caused users to eat fewer calories.[27] Also, 5-HTP helps some individuals alleviate insomnia. And 5-HTP helps depression, which could reduce emotional eating due to depressed moods such as sadness, loneliness, and self-loathing.

Maca powder

Maca is an annual plant grown in Peru that produces a radish-like root. The Peruvians claim that Maca increases energy, helps depression and anemia, and improves overall memory and vitality. This powerful food is also a libido stimulant! More energy equates to more activity and burning more calories.

Inulin

Inulin is a low-glycemic, soluble fiber that assumes a gel-like consistency when exposed to water. Inulin increases satiety—the sensation of fullness. It's found in sunchokes (Jerusalem artichokes), asparagus stems, chicory root (used most often to make commercial inulin), artichoke bulb, and salsify root. This fiber cuts your craving for food. Also, the probiotic nature of inulin helps provide an environment for healthy bacteria to continue growing in the intestinal tract. A study with children published in the *Journal of Pediatrics* showed that supplements of inulin resulted in a much lower body mass index (BMI) over a one-year period.[28]

Chapter 8

The Turbo Diet Meal Plan

THE MEAL PLANS in this chapter are designed to help you lose the maximum weight you can in the healthiest possible way. To that end, the menu plan with raw foods is placed first. It's positioned before the plan that includes cooked vegan and animal products so you can try a mostly raw foods diet for a week or two, if you like, to give you the best jump start for your weight-loss plan. Though you can alternately use the menu plan that incorporates more cooked food and animal products, keep in mind that raw foods work so well for weight loss because these foods are loaded with enzymes, fiber, vitamins, minerals, and phytonutrients. The enzymes spare your liver and pancreas, which produce digestive juices, and frees up these organs to concentrate on other work. The fiber helps carry fat out of your body. And the abundance of antioxidants and other nutrients found in the juices curb your cravings and help detoxify your entire system.

Supporting the liver is very important in a weight-loss program because it is the major fat-burning organ of the body and regulates fat metabolism. It can also pump excess fat out of the body through the bile into the small intestines. When the diet is high in fiber and nutrients, this unwanted fat will be carried away. A healthy liver is a remarkable organ for keeping weight under control since it's both a fat-burning and a fat-pumping organ. The Turbo Diet Raw Foods Menu Plan is especially rich in fiber and nutrients to give your liver the tools it needs for a great kick start to weight loss.

The delicious recipes and menu suggestions in this chapter provide plenty of ideas for ways to incorporate more live foods into your food plan and maximize your weight-loss potential.

TURBO DIET KITCHEN EQUIPMENT
RECOMMENDATIONS

There are several kitchen equipment items that will make your food preparation much easier on the Turbo Diet. A juicer and blender are very helpful to own, and the other items will help you make great food you can enjoy so that you will be more inclined to stick with your Turbo Diet Weight-Loss Plan.

- **Juicer.** A good juicer that is easy to use and clean is the main tool in your Turbo Diet. If you don't have a juicer or are unhappy with the one you have, and you're wondering which juicer is right for you, see chapter 2 on choosing a juicer. Also, check Appendix A for additional information.
- **Blender.** A blender is needed to make the great raw soups and savory smoothie recipes in chapter 9. But you don't have to spend a lot of money to get a good blender. Most blenders work just fine. The top of the line is the Vita Mix, which does a tremendous job.
- **Dehydrator.** Though a dehydrator is not necessary to make the Turbo Diet work, it's a great appliance that enables you to make delicious low-calorie, low-glycemic snacks that will make this diet enjoyable and easy. Check out Appendix A for recommendations.
- **Spiral slicer or spirooli slicer.** The spiral slicer, originally from Japan, is used to make raw spaghetti dishes, thin slices for dehydrated veggies, and curls for decorative salads and dishes. (The spaghetti is more like linguini width with the spiral slicer.) The spirooli is a three-in-one turning slicer for vegetables; it slices, shreds, and chips veggies on a rotating arm. It makes a thicker strand than the spiral slicer—more like spaghetti width. You can turn almost any vegetable into spaghetti-type strands, slices, or julienne strips, such as onion, zucchini, carrot, cucumber, turnip, potato, sweet potato, daikon radish, and butternut squash.
- **Mandolin food slicer** makes crinkle cuts, thin uniform slices, and julienne strips in a variety of thicknesses. The blade ensures even soft foods like tomatoes slice

perfectly. This tool is very helpful to make thin slices for dehydrated foods and raw dishes.

Fast-Track Weight-Loss Tips

Following these tips will propel your weight-loss success with a great kick start.

- Drink a minimum of two 10- to 12-ounce glasses of vegetable juice every day.
- For the best success, strive to eat between 75 and 80 percent of your foods raw. (Foods that have been dehydrated at 105 degrees are considered raw because the enzymes and vitamins have not been destroyed with heat.)
- For at least the first three weeks, omit all starchy vegetables such as potatoes, yams, winter squash, corn, and peas. Also, omit all grains. You can have wild rice; it's actually a cereal grass and is lower in carbohydrates.
- Limit nuts for snacks to no more than a dozen per day and seeds to no more than 1 or 2 tablespoons; nut butters to about 1 teaspoon. Nuts contain carbohydrates.
- Make one day a week a juice feast day. On this day, consume only vegetable juices and raw soups along with the water quota and green, white, or herbal tea.
- Drink eight to ten glasses of purified water every day. If you add a little cranberry juice or cranberry concentrate to the water, it will help to flush fat and will also act as a diuretic. Buy pure, unsweetened cranberry juice or cranberry juice concentrate. This also helps to curb your appetite.
- Have a small snack or glass of vegetable juice in the midmorning and midafternoon. This will help to keep your blood sugar stable so that you won't be tempted to overeat at lunch or eat snack foods before dinner or overeat at your evening meal.
- The lighter the evening meal, the faster you will lose weight, because we don't typically burn as many calories in the evening as we do during the day.
- Develop an exercise plan that includes a varied workout three to four times a week.

THE FAST TRACK ONE-DAY JUICE DIET

To accelerate your weight loss, include the One-Day Vegetable Juice Diet each week. You could pick a day you are off from work to make this easier for you, but you can also juice ahead and take your juice to work. This is an all-liquid day that helps you detox your body and flush out fat. During this day, you will only drink vegetable juice, vegetable broth, water, sparkling mineral water, and herbal, green, or white teas. If you find that you are too spacey or your blood sugar drops too low, add a bowl of raw energy soup for one meal. This day is a great boost to weight loss! It will especially help you get rid of stored-up water and toxins while at the same time rejuvenating your body.

Breakfast
- Green, white, or herbal tea with lemon juice or hot water with lemon and a dash of cayenne pepper (this helps the liver get moving)
- Vegetable juice recipe of choice

Midmorning
- 9:30 a.m.: 8 ounces of water or cranberry water
- 10:30 a.m.: Vegetable juice of choice
- 11:30 a.m.: Green, white, or herbal tea or 8 ounces of water or sparkling mineral water*

Lunch
- Vegetable juice recipe of choice

Midafternoon
- 1:30 p.m.: 8 ounces water or cranberry water
- 2:30 p.m.: 8 ounces water or cranberry water
- 3:00 p.m.: Vegetable juice of choice
- 4:00 p.m.: 8 ounces water or cranberry water
- 5:00 p.m.: 8 ounces water or cranberry water

Dinner
- Vegetable juice of choice
- (You may also add a cup of warm vegetable broth.)

---

* Sparkling mineral water may be substituted for water at any time. You may add a squeeze of lemon or lime for added flavor, or unsweetened cranberry juice.

Menu Plan with Raw and Some Cooked Vegan Foods

There are two menu plans in this section—the all-raw menu plan and a menu plan with some cooked vegan foods and some animal products. You can adapt either menu plan to fit your needs.

You will drink two glasses of vegetable juice each day. Make fresh juice whenever you can. If you can't make fresh juice, you can buy it at a juice bar. Or you can get refrigerated juice or low-sodium V-8. You may have more than two glasses of vegetable juice a day, but not less. The time of day you drink the juice is up to you. Many people like to start their day with fresh juice to energize their mind and body, while others take juice to work in a stainless steel water bottle or thermos and drink it midmorning as a pick-me-up. The other glass of juice should be consumed either midafternoon or before dinner. This will help to curb your appetite so that you will eat less at dinner and not be tempted to snack before or after dinner. The evening meal should be light since evening is the time when most of us get the least exercise and burn the fewest number of calories. If this schedule does not work well for your lifestyle, then fit the glasses of veggie juice in where you can. The following menu plan is simply a guideline to help you see how you can plan your days. You can use the recipes and ideas in this chapter or choose your own that fit the low-glycemic guidelines for healthy eating. Remember, that means keep the refined and starchy carbohydrates out of your diet and completely avoid refined and processed foods.

A juice of choice is listed for breakfast with a juice of choice as optional midmorning. The same goes for the afternoon. This does not mean you need to drink two glasses of juice in the morning and two glasses in the afternoon, unless you desire; the options are there so you can choose the time that fits best. And recipes are listed just to give you an idea of the recipes available to you. This in no way means that you have to drink that recipe at that time. Choose the recipes you like, and fit them into your menu plan.

Day 1

Breakfast
- Juice of choice, such as The Morning Energizer (page 172)

- Cherie's Awesome Green Smoothie with ground almonds (page 181)
- Green, white, or herbal tea (and a squeeze of lemon is nice)

Midmorning snack
- Juice of choice (optional)
- Granny Smith or pippin apple

Lunch
- Refreshing Salsa Shake (page 189)
- 1 Corn Cracker (page 198)

Midafternoon snack
- Juice of choice (optional)
- Veggie sticks

Dinner
- Juice of choice, such as Super Green Drink (page 173)
- Dinner salad with dressing of choice
- South of the Border Lettuce Wraps (page 205)

Day 2

Breakfast
- Juice of choice, such as Spicy Pink Morning (page 177)
- Green, white, or herbal tea (and a squeeze of lemon is nice)
- Sprouted Buckwheat Groats (page 200) with almond, oat, or rice milk, 1 tablespoon ground almonds, and a dash of cinnamon (optional)

Midmorning snack
- Juice of choice (optional)
- Veggie sticks

Lunch
- Creamy Tomato Soup (page 186)
- Spring greens with Lemon Vinaigrette (page 202)

Midafternoon snack
- Juice of choice (optional)
- 1 Broccoli Latkes (page 197)

Dinner
- Juice of choice, such as Jicama Surprise (page 173)
- Asian Salad (page 203)
- 1 Garlicky Jicama Cracker (page 198)

Day 3

Breakfast
- Juice of choice, such as Happy Mood Morning (page 167)
- The Health Nut Smoothie (page 185)
- Green, white, or herbal tea (and a squeeze of lemon is nice)

Midmorning snack
- Juice of choice (optional)
- Half dozen sun-dried or naturally processed green or black organic olives

Lunch
- French Tomato Basil Soup (page 188)
- 1 Veggie Cracker

Midafternoon snack
- Juice of choice (optional)
- 4 Kale Chips (page 195)

Dinner
- Juice of choice, such as Spicy Tomato (page 170)
- Mixed green salad with your favorite dressing
- Stuffed Bell Peppers (page 205)

Day 4

Breakfast
- Juice of choice, such as Mood Mender (page 172)
- Guilt-Free "Bacon" (page 199)
- Sliced tomatoes or sliced avocado
- Green, white, or herbal tea (and a squeeze of lemon is nice)

Midmorning snack
- Juice of choice (optional)
- Celery sticks with 1 teaspoon almond butter

Lunch
- Quick Energy Soup (page 181)
- Sliced tomatoes with extra-virgin olive oil and balsamic vinegar
- 1 Seed Cracker (page 199)

Midafternoon snack
- Juice of choice (optional)
- Dehydrated Onion Rings (page 196)

Dinner
- Juice of choice, such as Mint Refresher (page 172)
- Sliced cucumbers with brown rice vinegar
- Easy Phad Thai (page 207)

Day 5

Breakfast
- Juice of choice, such as Have a Great Day Cocktail (page 162)
- Sprouted rye cereal (page 200) with oat, almond, or rice milk and ground almonds, as desired
- Fresh or frozen berries: blueberries, blackberries, or strawberries
- Green, white, or herbal tea (and a squeeze of lemon is nice)

Midmorning snack
- Juice of choice (optional)
- 2 tablespoons sunflower seeds

Lunch
- Eggless Salad Roll-ups (page 203)
- 1 Veggie Cracker (page 198)

Midafternoon snack
- Juice of choice (optional)
- 3–4 Dehydrated Tomatoes and Basil (page 196)

Dinner
- Juice of choice, such as Beet-Ginger Cleansing Cocktail (page 163)
- Jalapeño Nut Burgers (page 206)

- Sliced tomatoes or Dehydrated Tomatoes and Basil (page 196)
- Green Salad with Lemon Tahini Dressing

Day 6

Breakfast
- Juice of choice, such as The Ginger Hopper (page 177)
- Sprouted rye bread* with raw almond butter
- Green, white, or herbal tea (and a squeeze of lemon is nice)

Midmorning snack
- Juice of choice (optional)
- Granny Smith or pippin apple or veggie sticks

Lunch
- Spinach salad with Lemon Vinaigrette (page 202)
- Yummy Yam Bisque (page 184)

Midafternoon break
- Juice of choice (optional)
- 6 raw almonds

Dinner
- Juice of choice, such as South of the Border Cocktail (page 175)
- Raw Enchiladas (page 208)
- Sliced tomatoes with extra-virgin olive oil and balsamic vinegar

Day 7

Breakfast
- Juice of choice, such as Twisted Ginger (page 167)
- The Health Nut Smoothie (page 185)
- Green, white, or herbal tea (and a squeeze of lemon is nice)

Midmorning snack
- Juice of choice (optional)
- Dehydrated Onion Rings (page 196)

Lunch
- Garden salad with Lemon Tahini Dressing
- Icy Spicy Gazpacho (page 183)

Midafternoon snack
- Juice of choice (optional)
- 1 Granny Smith or pippin apple

Dinner
- Juice of choice, such as Weight-Loss Buddy (page 180)
- Spicy Peanut Sauce over Zucchini Noodles (page 206)

MENU PLAN WITH SOME COOKED VEGAN FOODS AND FISH AND CHICKEN DISHES

Day 1

Breakfast
- Juice of choice, such as The Ginger Hopper (page 177)
- Cherie's Awesome Green Smoothie with ground almonds (page 181)
- Green, white, or herbal tea (and a squeeze of lemon is nice)

Midmorning snack
- Juice of choice (optional)
- 4 Kale Chips (page 195)

Lunch
- Chipotle Bean Soup (page 214)
- Coleslaw or Caesar salad

Midafternoon snack
- Juice of choice (optional)
- 2 tablespoons raw sunflower or pumpkin seeds

Dinner
- Juice of choice, such as Weight-Loss Buddy (page 180)
- Dinner salad with Lemon-Tarragon Vinaigrette (page 202)
- Springtime Vegetables with Cashew-Carrot Sauce (page 213)

Day 2

Breakfast
- Juice of choice, such as Happy Mood Morning (page 167)
- Green, white, or herbal tea (and a squeeze of lemon is nice)
- Sprouted Buckwheat Groats (page 200) with almond, oat, or rice milk and cinnamon and sprinkle of ground nuts, as desired *or*
- Oatmeal with almond, oat, or rice milk

Midmorning snack
- Veggie sticks with 1 tablespoon of hummus

Lunch
- Grilled Chicken or Salmon Caesar Salad
- 1 Veggie Cracker (page 198)

Midafternoon snack
- Juice of choice (optional)
- 6 raw almonds

Dinner
- Juice of choice, such as Super Green Drink (page 173)
- Cashew Vegetable Curry (page 217)
- 1/2 cup wild rice
- Green salad with Lemon Vinaigrette

Day 3

Breakfast
- Juice of choice, such as The Morning Energizer (page 172)
- The Health Nut Smoothie (page 185)
- Green, white, or herbal tea (and a squeeze of lemon is nice)

Midmorning snack
- Juice of choice (optional)
- 1 Broccoli Latkes (page 197)

Lunch
- Mixed green salad with dressing of choice

- Summer Corn Chowder (page 186) or Refreshing Cucumber-Mint Soup (page 186)
- 1 Corn Cracker (page 198)

Midafternoon snack
- Juice of choice (optional)
- 6 raw almonds

Dinner
- Juice of choice, such as Spicy Tomato (page 170)
- South of the Border Lettuce Wraps (page 205)
- Sliced tomatoes with fresh basil and balsamic vinegar

Day 4

Breakfast
- Juice of choice, such as Spicy Pink Morning (page 177)
- 3 ounces broiled or smoked salmon
- Sliced tomatoes or sliced avocado
- Green, white, or herbal tea (and a squeeze of lemon is nice)

Midmorning snack
- 4 celery sticks and radishes or carrot sticks
- 1 Garlicky Jicama Cracker (page 198)

Lunch
- Moroccan Stew (page 214) or Red Lentil Spinach Soup (page 216)
- Sliced tomatoes with extra-virgin olive oil and balsamic vinegar

Midafternoon snack
- Juice of choice (optional)
- Half dozen sun-dried or naturally processed green or black organic olives

Dinner
- Juice of choice, such as Green Refresher (page 160)
- Garlic Dijon Halibut (page 221)
- Steamed vegetable such as broccoli or brussels sprouts
- Green salad with dressing of choice

Day 5

Breakfast

- Juice of choice, such as Mood Mender (page 172)
- 1 boiled egg
- Sliced tomatoes with chopped fresh (or dried) basil
- Green, white, or herbal tea (and a squeeze of lemon is nice)

Midmorning snack

- Juice of choice (optional)
- 2 tablespoons sunflower seeds

Lunch

- Salad greens with Lemon–Olive Oil Dressing
- Sunshine "Eggless" Salad Roll-ups (page 203) or salmon salad roll-ups

Midafternoon snack

- Juice of choice (optional)
- Dehydrated Onion Rings (page 196)

Dinner

- Juice of choice, such as Parsley Patch (page 160)
- Garden salad with Lemon Tahini Dressing
- Steamed vegetable such as green beans or broccoli
- Moroccan Chicken with Lemon and Olives (page 220)

Day 6

Breakfast

- Juice of choice, such as Have a Great Day Cocktail (page 162)
- Sprouted rye bread with raw almond butter
- Green, white, or herbal tea (and a squeeze of lemon is nice)

Midmorning snack

- Juice of choice (optional)
- Granny Smith or pippin apple or veggie sticks

Lunch
- Yummy Yam Bisque (page 184)
- Green salad with dressing of choice

Midafternoon snack
- Juice of choice (optional)
- Dehydrated Tomatoes and Basil (page 196)

Dinner
- Juice of choice, such as South of the Border Cocktail (page 175)
- Raw Enchiladas (page 208)
- Garden salad with dressing of choice (page 202)

Day 7

Breakfast
- Juice of choice, such as Magnesium-Rich Cocktail (page 171)
- Cherie's Awesome Green Smoothie with ground almonds (page 181)
- Green, white, or herbal tea (and a squeeze of lemon is nice)

Midmorning snack
- 1 slice of turkey
- Radishes and cucumber slices

Lunch
- Green salad with dressing of choice
- Jalapeño Nut Burgers (page 206) or veggie burger with sliced tomatoes

Midafternoon snack
- Juice of choice (optional)
- 1 Veggie Cracker (page 198)

Dinner
- Juice of choice, such as Beet-Ginger Cleansing Cocktail (page 163)
- Chicken Curry (page 220)
- Caesar or spinach salad with dressing of choice

SET YOUR GOALS; KEEP TRACK OF YOUR ACTIONS

In getting started, it's important to keep track of the foods you eat each day. At the end of this chapter is a daily food diary; you can make copies of this diary and fill it out each day. Write down everything you eat. Sometimes we don't realize all we are eating until we write it down, because we take a bite of something and forget about it or we grab a few nuts or a snack item at work, pop them in our mouth, and off we go! It's the small things that add up fast and often derail us from our track. It's important to note everything you eat so you can make changes that are helpful to achieve your goals.

Every day take inventory. Are you drinking the water you need for optimal weight loss? How about green or white tea, which has thermogenic effects? Are you drinking two glasses of vegetable juice each day? What food choices did you make? Were three-quarters of the food you ate raw? How much food did you eat in the evening? If you look at what you're doing objectively, you can make adjustments that will move you forward.

SET YOUR GOALS

There's a quote I read often: "To get something you never had, you have to do something you never did." You know what they say about those people who keep doing the same thing over and over again and expect different results—that's insanity! One definition of insanity is *extreme foolishness*. To become a new you, you must see yourself in a new way—as the person you choose to become—and adopt new action steps. You will succeed by choosing outcome-based behaviors you haven't done consistently before.

Though I've talked about weight loss throughout this book, when you set your goals, it's helpful to reframe that to what you want to weigh by the end of the first week, the end of the month, then the end of the year. Write those goals down. The goal of losing or weight loss may not take you in the direction you want to go, but the goal of choosing what you want to weigh, what you want to achieve, can be powerful. See yourself as the thinner, trimmer self you choose to become with your interior eyes. This is a compelling action to achieve the right outcome. So rather than loss, you can have achievement, success, a trimmer body, and better health.

Close your eyes for a moment. Can you see yourself at your ideal

weight? Now decide, realistically, what you would like to weigh by the
end of the first week on the Turbo Diet.

- Week one I want to weigh _____.
- Week two I want to weigh _____.
- Week three I want to weigh _____.
- Week four I want to weigh _____.
- Now, write down your goal weight for each week after
  that and see yourself achieving your goal. Also, write
  down your goals for exercise—how many times will
  you exercise a week, and what type of workouts will
  you do?

Start a goal-minded picture board. Cut out a picture of a person
that resembles the weight you want to achieve. Put it up in a place
where you can see it often. This storyboard of goals does work. I did
a storyboard of pictures years ago when I set my career goals. I still
display it in my office. I had a picture of a writer on the page with a
goal of writing many books. At the time I had only co-written one
book. *The Juice Lady's Turbo Diet* is book number seventeen. I put
a picture of a television on there because I wanted to do something
in my field on TV since my undergrad degree is in speech communications. To date, I've been on hundreds of talk and news shows,
have made appearances in five infomercials, and have appeared on
QVC regularly for thirteen years with the George Foreman grills
and the Juiceman and Juice Lady Juicers. So as you can see, setting
pictures before your eyes can have a tremendous influence on your
outcome.

As you set your goals, tack up your storyboard where you can see it,
and embark on your weight-reduction journey, keep a positive mental
attitude. Tell yourself each day that you can do this. You can achieve
your goals. Praise yourself often for all the right choices you make.
Don't beat yourself up for the mistakes. You can become a new you.
You can fulfill the purpose for your life in the trim, fit body that will
best help you run your unique race of life.

Please know that I'm in your corner. I'm cheering for you. My
prayers are with you. I want to hear your story—your small successes
and your great ones. Don't ever give up. Remember that I didn't.
Through all the obstacles, tragedies, and trials you read about in

chapter 6, I just kept going. And I'm here today, by a series of miracles and a lot of hard work, living my dream and doing my best to help you. You can do it too. One day, just like so many other people I've worked with, you will be standing in your dream and living your life to its zenith!

Daily Food Diary for the Juice Lady's Turbo Diet

Day _____

Vegetable juice and other liquids
- Glass 1 _____
- Glass 2 _____
- Water (minimum eight 8-ounce glasses per day)
  _____
- Herbal tea _____
- Green tea _____

Supplements
- _____
- _____

Foods
- Grains _____
- Vegetables _____
- Fruit _____
- Meat/fish/poultry _____
- Fats _____
- Other _____

DIET DIARY

Breakfast	
Midmorning snack	
Lunch	
Midafternoon snack	
Dinner	

Chapter 9

The Turbo Diet Recipes

THE JUICE RECIPES in this chapter are designed to be low glycemic. To achieve that end, there is very little fruit used in the recipes. Most of them use lime or lemon (very low in sugar, very alkaline in their final breakdown) for flavor. You might want to try Meyer lemons in your recipes since they are sweeter. You can add ½ to 1 whole apple to any of the recipes to improve the flavor as well. Green apples are lower in sugar than red or yellow and a good choice for the low-glycemic diet. Carrots and beets are higher in sugar than other vegetables, but carrots are still in the low-glycemic category and beets are in the moderate category. They both offer excellent health benefits; therefore, I don't suggest omitting them unless they adversely affect you. You can dilute the sugars by adding very low-sugar vegetables such as cucumber, celery, and kale to your recipes.

Green Refresher

> 1 medium to large organic cucumber, peeled if not
>   organic
> 1 large leaf of green kale
> 1-2 stalks celery
> 1 lemon or lime, peeled

Cut produce to fit your juicer's feed tube. Juice ingredients and stir. Pour into a glass and drink as soon as possible. Serves 1.

Parsley Patch

> 1 handful parsley
> 1 lemon, peeled
> 2 carrots, scrubbed well, tops removed, ends trimmed
> 1-2 stalks celery with leaves
> 1 cucumber, peeled if not organic

Cut produce to fit your juicer's feed tube. Bunch up parsley and add to the juicer before turning it on. Then add lemon and place the plunger in place. Turn on the machine and juice remaining ingredients. Stir, then pour into a glass. Drink as soon as possible. Serves 2.

Antiulcer Cabbage Cocktail

Scientific research has proven that cabbage juice is an effective treatment for stomach ulcers.

> ¼ small head green cabbage
> 3 carrots, scrubbed well, tops removed, ends trimmed
> 4 celery stalks, with leaves if desired

Cut produce to fit your juicer's feed tube. Juice ingredients and stir. Pour into a glass and drink as soon as possible. Serves 1.

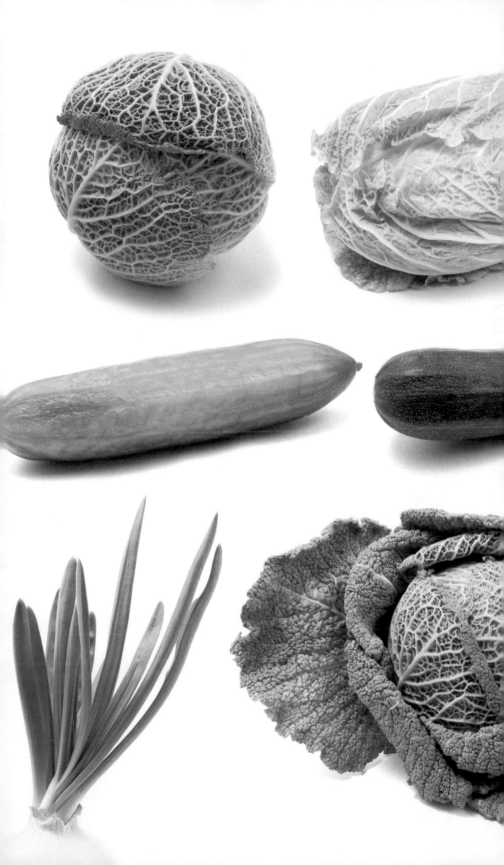

Antiviral Cocktail

> 4–5 carrots, scrubbed well, tops removed, ends trimmed
> ½ cucumber, peeled if not organic
> 1 garlic clove with peel
> 1 small turnip, scrubbed well
> 1 handful watercress, rinsed
> 1 lemon, peeled

Cut produce to fit your juicer's feed tube. Juice ingredients and stir. Pour into a glass and drink as soon as possible. Serves 1–2.

Have a Great Day Cocktail

> 1 green apple
> 1–2 kale leaves
> 1 handful parsley
> 1 stalk celery with leaves, as desired
> 1 lemon, peeled
> ½ cucumber, peeled if not organic
> ½- to 1-inch piece fresh gingerroot, peeled

Cut the apple into sections that fit your juicer's feed tube. Bunch up the kale and parsley, and push through the feed tube with the apple, celery, lemon, cucumber, and ginger. Stir the juice, and pour into a glass. Serve at room temperature or chilled, as desired. Serves 1–2.

Antiaging Cocktail

Parsnips, cucumber, and bell pepper are good sources of the trace mineral silicon, which is recommended to strengthen skin, hair, and fingernails as well as bones. In studies, silicon has been shown to reduce signs of aging by improving thickness of skin and reducing wrinkles.

> 2–3 carrots, scrubbed well, tops removed, ends trimmed
> 1 cucumber, peeled if not organic
> 1 small parsnip
> 1 lemon, peeled
> ¼ green bell pepper

Cut produce to fit your juicer's feed tube. Juice ingredients and stir. Pour into a glass and drink as soon as possible. Serves 1–2.

Beet-Ginger Cleansing Cocktail

3 carrots, scrubbed well, tops removed, ends trimmed
1 cucumber, peeled if not organic
1 beet with stem and leaves, scrubbed well
2 stalks celery
1 handful parsley
1- to 2-inch chunk gingerroot, scrubbed or peeled
1 lemon, peeled

Cut produce to fit your juicer's feed tube. Juice all ingredients and stir. Pour into a glass and drink as soon as possible. Serves 1–2.

Natural Diuretic Tonic

Cucumber, asparagus, and lemon are all natural diuretics. Getting rid of old stored-up water is a great boost to your weight-loss program.

1 medium vine-ripened tomato
1 organic cucumber, peeled if not organic
8 asparagus stems
1 lemon or lime, peeled
Dash of hot sauce

Cut produce to fit your juicer's feed tube. Juice all ingredients except hot sauce. Pour into a glass, stir in hot sauce, and drink as soon as possible. Serves 1–2.

The Cabbage Patch

3 stalks celery with leaves
3 carrots, scrubbed well, tops removed, ends trimmed
1 tomato
1 lemon, peeled
¼ green cabbage (spring or summer cabbage is best)

Cut produce to fit your juicer's feed tube. Juice ingredients and stir. Pour into a glass and drink as soon as possible. Serves 1.

Calcium-Plus Cocktail

Kale and parsley are loaded with calcium, but that's not all. They also have magnesium, boron, and vitamin K—all are important for bone health.

1 cucumber, peeled if not organic
1 large kale leaf
1 handful parsley
1 celery stalk
1 lemon, peeled
1-inch chunk gingerroot, scrubbed or peeled if old

Cut produce to fit your juicer's feed tube. Juice ingredients and stir. Pour into a glass and drink as soon as possible. Serves 1–2.

Happy Colon Tonic

Apples are a good source of soluble fiber, which is very good for color health. There is soluble fiber in juice.

1 green apple
1 cucumber, peeled if not organic
1 lemon, peeled
1 handful spinach
1 handful parsley

Cut produce to fit your juicer's feed tube. Juice ingredients and stir. Pour into a glass and drink as soon as possible. Serves 1.

Cran-Apple Cocktail

2 organic green apples
¼–½ cup fresh or frozen (thawed) cranberries
½ lemon, peeled
1-inch chunk gingerroot
¼ cup purified water (optional)

Cut produce to fit your juicer's feed tube. Juice 1 apple first. Turn off the machine, add the cranberries, put the plunger in, then turn the machine on and juice. Follow with the lemon, ginger, and second apple. Add water as needed. Stir and pour into a glass; drink as soon as possible. Serves 1–2.

Gallbladder Cleansing Cocktail

Carrots and beets are considered cleansing vegetables for the gallbladder.

1 cucumber, peeled if not organic
1 lemon, peeled
5 carrots, scrubbed well, tops removed, ends trimmed
1 small to medium beet with leaves and stems,
    scrubbed well

Cut produce to fit your juicer's feed tube. Juice ingredients and stir. Pour into a glass and drink as soon as possible. Serves 1.

Liver-Gallbladder Rejuvenator

Cabbage, citrus fruits, and lemon peel oils stimulate the liver. Beet and carrot juice are rejuvenating for the liver.

3-4 carrots, scrubbed well, tops removed, ends trimmed
1 chunk purple cabbage
1 lemon
½ beet with leaves and stems, scrubbed well
1-inch piece ginger
½ green apple (optional)

Cut produce to fit your juicer's feed tube. Juice ingredients and stir. Pour into a glass and drink as soon as possible. Serves 1-2.

Garlic Wonder

Handful parsley
1 dark green lettuce leaf such as green leaf or romaine
½ cucumber, peeled
1 garlic clove
3 carrots, scrubbed well, tops removed, ends trimmed
2 stalks celery with leaves, as desired

Roll the parsley in the lettuce leaf. Juice the cucumber, then the parsley rolled in the lettuce leaf. Add the garlic and push through the juicer with the carrots, followed by the celery. Stir and pour into a glass. Serves 1-2.

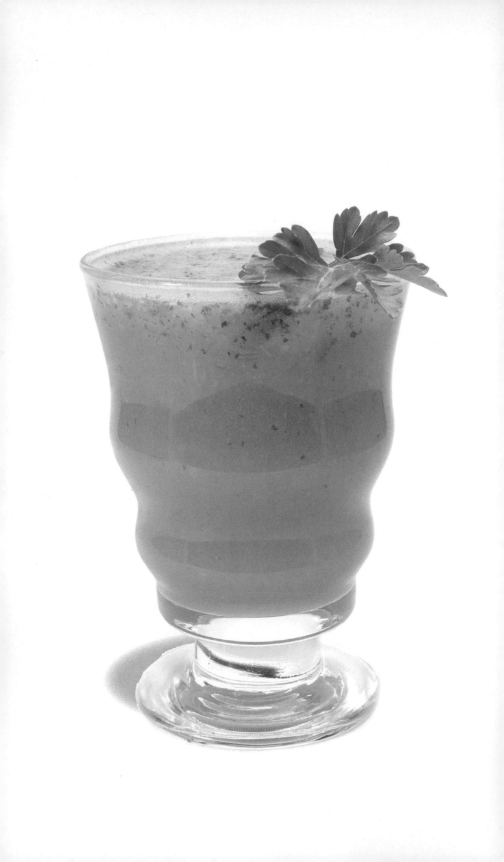

Twisted Ginger

4 carrots, scrubbed well, tops removed, ends trimmed
1 handful parsley
1 lemon, peeled
1 apple
2-inch piece fresh gingerroot, peeled

Cut produce to fit your juicer's feed tube. Juice ingredients and stir. Pour into a glass and drink as soon as possible. Serves 1–2.

The Gout Fighter

A 1950 study of twelve individuals with gout showed that eating ½ pound of cherries or drinking the equivalent amount of cherry juice prevented gout attacks. Black, sweet yellow, and red sour cherries were all effective.[1]

1 green apple
½ pound cherries, pits removed
2 stalks celery with leaves, as desired
1 lemon, peeled if not organic

Cut produce to fit your juicer's feed tube. Juice ingredients and stir. Pour into a glass and drink as soon as possible. Serves 1.

Happy Mood Morning

Fennel juice has been used as a traditional tonic to help the body release endorphins, the "feel-good" peptides, from the brain into the bloodstream. Endorphins help to diminish anxiety and fear and generate a mood of euphoria.

½ green apple
4–5 carrots, well scrubbed, tops removed, ends trimmed
3 fennel stalks; include leaves and flowers
½ cucumber
Handful spinach
1-inch piece gingerroot

Cut produce to fit your juicer's feed tube. Juice apple first and follow with other ingredients. Stir and pour into a glass; drink as soon as possible. Serves 1.

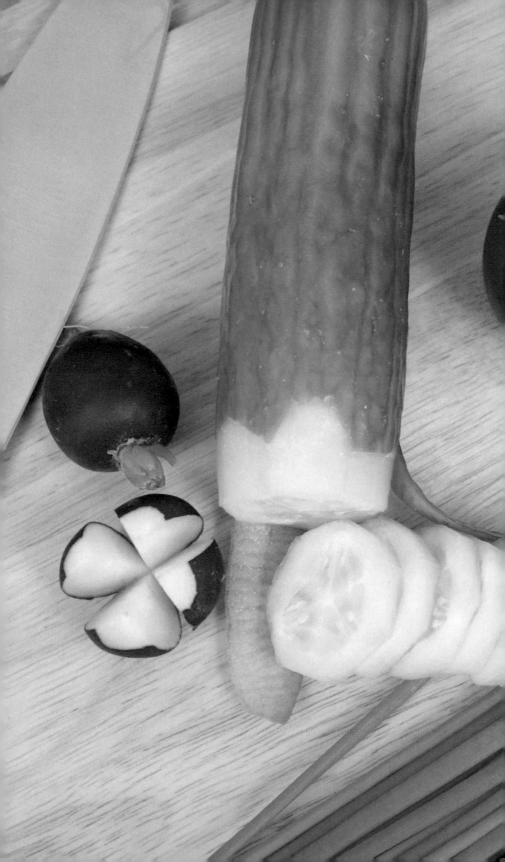

Lung Rejuvenator

Turnip juice has been used as a traditional remedy to strengthen lung tissue.

  1 handful watercress
  1 small turnip, scrubbed well, tops removed, ends
    trimmed
  2-inch thick chunk of jicama, scrubbed well or peeled
  1 garlic clove
  ½ lemon, peeled
  2-3 carrots, scrubbed well, tops removed, ends trimmed

Bunch up watercress. Cut produce to fit your juicer's feed tube. Tuck the watercress in feed tube and push through with the turnip. Juice remaining ingredients, finishing with carrots. Stir the juice, pour into a glass, and drink as soon as possible. Serves 1.

Healthy Sinus Solution

Radish juice is a traditional remedy to open up the sinuses and support mucous membranes.

  2 tomatoes
  6 radishes
  1 lime, peeled
  ½ cucumber, peeled if not organic

Cut produce to fit your juicer's feed tube. Juice ingredients and stir. Pour into a glass and drink as soon as possible. Serves 1.

Immune Builder

Studies show that garlic has allicin, a compound with a natural antibiotic-like effect. It is antibacterial, antifungal, antiparasitic, and antiviral, but it must be consumed raw to have this effect.

1 handful watercress
1 turnip, scrubbed, tops removed, ends trimmed
3 carrots, scrubbed well, tops removed, ends trimmed
1–2 garlic cloves
½ green apple such as Granny Smith or pippin
1 lemon, peeled

Bunch up watercress. Cut produce to fit your juicer's feed tube. Tuck the watercress in feed tube and push through with the turnip. Finish with remaining ingredients. Stir the juice, pour into a glass, and drink as soon as possible. Serves 1.

Spicy Tomato

2 medium tomatoes
2 dark green lettuce leaves
2 radishes
Small handful of parsley
1 lime or lemon, peeled
Dash of hot sauce

Cut produce to fit your juicer's feed tube. Juice ingredients and stir. Pour into a glass and drink as soon as possible. Serves 1.

Pancreas Helper

Brussels sprouts and string bean juice have been used as traditional remedies to help strengthen and support the pancreas. Drink before a meal. (If this drink is too strong, dilute with a little water.)

1 large tomato
2 romaine lettuce leaves
8 string beans
2 brussels sprouts
1 lemon, peeled

Cut produce to fit your juicer's feed tube. Juice ingredients and stir. Pour into a glass and drink as soon as possible. Serves 1.

Liver Life Tonic

Dandelion juice is a traditional remedy for cleansing the liver.

1 handful of dandelion greens
3–4 carrots, scrubbed well, tops removed, ends trimmed
1 cucumber, peeled if not organic
1 lemon, peeled

Bunch up dandelion greens. Cut produce to fit your juicer's feed tube. Tuck the greens in feed tube and push through with a carrot. Juice the remaining ingredients. Stir the juice, pour into a glass, and drink as soon as possible. Serves 1.

Magnesium-Rich Cocktail

3–4 carrots, scrubbed well, tops removed, ends trimmed
2–3 broccoli florets
2 celery stalks, with leaves as desired
½ small beet, scrubbed well
½ lemon, peeled

Cut produce to fit your juicer's feed tube. Juice ingredients and stir. Pour into a glass and drink as soon as possible. Serves 1.

Memory Tonic

Broccoli, cauliflower, and brussels sprouts are all rich in choline, an essential nutrient for memory and brain health. Choline is a precursor to the neurotransmitter acetylcholine, which contributes to healthy and efficient brain processes.

2 medium tomatoes
1 lemon, peeled
1 green leaf lettuce
4 cauliflower florets, washed
1 garlic clove

Cut produce to fit your juicer's feed tube. Juice ingredients and stir. Pour into a glass and drink as soon as possible. Serves 1–2.

Mint Refresher

2 stalks fennel with leaves
1 cucumber, peeled if not organic
1 green apple such as Granny Smith or pippin
1 handful mint
1-inch chunk gingerroot, scrubbed or peeled if old

Cut produce to fit your juicer's feed tube. Juice ingredients and stir. Pour into a glass and drink as soon as possible. Serves 1–2.

Mood Mender

Fennel juice has been used as a traditional tonic to help the body release endorphins, the "feel-good" peptides, from the brain into the bloodstream. Endorphins help to diminish anxiety and fear and generate a mood of euphoria.

3 fennel stalks with leaves
3 carrots, scrubbed well, tops removed, ends trimmed
2 stalks celery with leaves, as desired
½ pear
1-inch chunk gingerroot, peeled

Cut produce to fit your juicer's feed tube. Juice ingredients and stir. Pour into a glass and drink as soon as possible. Serves 1–2.

The Morning Energizer

3–4 carrots, scrubbed well, tops removed, ends trimmed
1 cucumber, peeled if not organic
1 small beet, scrubbed well, with stems and leaves
1 lemon, peeled
1-inch chunk gingerroot, peeled
½ green apple

Cut produce to fit your juicer's feed tube. Juice all ingredients and stir. Pour into a glass and drink as soon as possible. Serves 1–2.

Jicama Surprise

2-inch by 4- or 5-inch chunk of jicama, scrubbed well or
　peeled
2–3 carrots, scrubbed well, tops removed, ends trimmed
½ cucumber, peeled if not organic
¼ daikon radish, trimmed and scrubbed
1-inch chunk gingerroot, scrubbed or peeled if old
½ lemon or lime, peeled

Cut produce to fit your juicer's feed tube. Juice ingredients and
stir. Pour into a glass and drink as soon as possible. Serves 1.

Allergy Relief

Parsley is a traditional remedy for allergic reactions. You need
to juice a bunch as soon as possible after a reaction occurs. It
can help open airways when sipped.

1 bunch parsley
2 celery stalks
1–2 carrots, scrubbed well, tops removed, ends trimmed
1 lemon, peeled
½ cucumber, peeled if not organic

Cut produce to fit your juicer's feed tube. Juice ingredients and
stir. Pour into a glass and drink as soon as possible. Serves 1.

Super Green Drink

1 cucumber, peeled if not organic
1 stalk celery with leaves, as desired
1 small handful sprouts such as broccoli or radish
1 large handful sunflower sprouts
1 small handful buckwheat sprouts
1 lemon, peeled

Cut produce to fit your juicer's feed tube. Juice ingredients and
stir. Pour into a glass and drink as soon as possible. Serves 1.

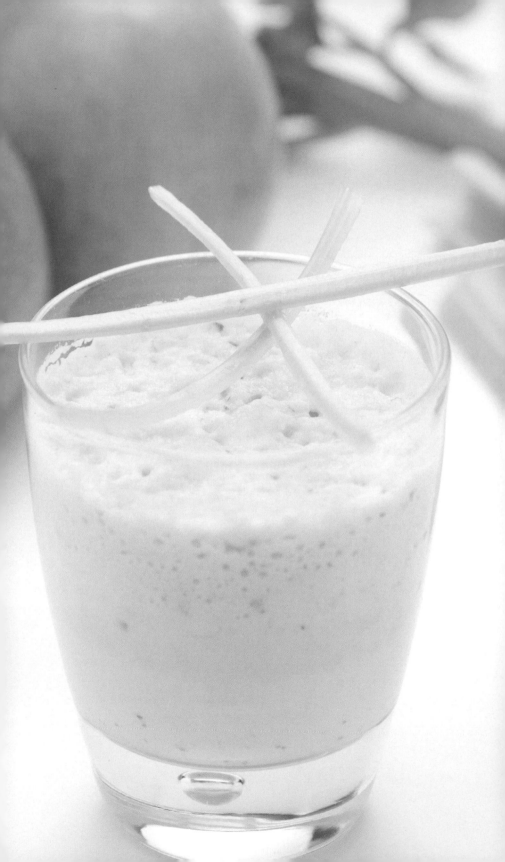

Radish Delight

> 5 carrots, scrubbed well, tops removed, ends trimmed
> 1 cucumber, peeled if not organic, or 1 large chunk of
>   jicama
> 5–6 radishes
> 1 lemon, peeled

Juice all the ingredients. Stir the juice and pour into a glass.
Serve at room temperature or chilled, as desired. Serves 1.

Root Veggie Cocktail

> 3–4 carrots, scrubbed well, tops removed, ends trimmed
> 1 cucumber, peeled
> ½ beet, scrubbed well, with stems and leaves
> ½ turnip, scrubbed
> 1 lemon, peeled
> ½ apple
> 1-inch chunk gingerroot, peeled

Cut produce to fit your juicer's feed tube. Juice all ingredients
and stir. Pour into a glass and drink as soon as possible.
Serves 1–2.

South of the Border Cocktail

> 1 medium tomato
> 1 cucumber, peeled if not organic
> 1 handful cilantro
> 1 lime, peeled
> Dash of hot sauce (optional)

Cut produce to fit your juicer's feed tube. Juice ingredients and
stir. Pour into a glass and drink as soon as possible. Serves 1.

Sleepytime Cocktail

Lettuce and celery help the body relax and help you sleep more deeply.

> 5 medium carrots, scrubbed well, tops removed, ends trimmed
> 2 stalks celery
> 2 romaine lettuce leaves
> 1 kale leaf
> 1 lemon, peeled
> ½ green apple, optional

Cut produce to fit your juicer's feed tube. Juice ingredients and stir. Pour into a glass and drink as soon as possible. Serves 1.

You Are Loved Cocktail

> 3 carrots, scrubbed well, tops removed, ends trimmed
> 2 celery stalks, with leaves
> 1 cucumber, peeled if not organic
> 1 handful spinach
> 1 lemon, peeled
> ½ beet, scrubbed well, with stems and leaves

Cut produce to fit your juicer's feed tube. Juice all ingredients and stir. Pour into a glass and drink as soon as possible. Serves 1–2.

Spring Veggie Tonic

Asparagus is a natural diuretic, which helps flush toxins from the body and promotes kidney cleansing. It's a great tonic for the kidneys. This recipe is a great way to use up asparagus stems.

> 1 tomato
> 1 cucumber, peeled if not organic
> 8 asparagus stems
> 1 lemon, peeled

Cut produce to fit your juicer's feed tube. Juice all ingredients and stir. Pour into a glass and drink as soon as possible. Serves 1–2.

Green Recharger

1 cucumber, peeled if not organic
1 handful sunflower sprouts
1 handful buckwheat sprouts
1 small handful clover sprouts (optional)
1 kale leaf
1 large handful spinach
1 lime, peeled

Cut the cucumber to fit your juicer's feed tube. Juice half of the cucumber first. Bunch up the sprouts and wrap in the kale leaf. Turn off the machine and add them. Turn the machine back on and tap with the rest of the cucumber to gently push the sprouts and kale through followed by spinach, and then juice the remaining cucumber and lime. Stir ingredients, pour into a glass, and drink as soon as possible. Serves 1.

Sweet Regularity

1 pear
1 apple
1 cucumber, peeled if not organic

Cut produce to fit your juicer's feed tube. Juice ingredients and stir. Pour into a glass and drink as soon as possible. Serves 1-2.

The Ginger Hopper

5 medium carrots, scrubbed well, tops removed, ends trimmed
1 green apple
1-inch piece fresh gingerroot, peeled

Cut produce to fit your juicer's feed tube. Juice ingredients and stir. Pour into a glass and drink as soon as possible. Serves 1.

Spicy Pink Morning

1 large pink grapefruit, peeled
1-inch piece fresh gingerroot, peeled

Cut produce to fit your juicer's feed tube. Juice ingredients and stir. Pour into a glass and drink as soon as possible. Serves 1.

The Pancreas Revitalizer

String beans are a traditional remedy for the pancreas. They are especially good for people with diabetes.

2 tomatoes
1 cucumber, peeled if not organic
6-8 string beans
1 lemon or lime, peeled
Dash of hot sauce

Cut produce to fit your juicer's feed tube. Juice ingredients, except for hot sauce. Add hot sauce and stir. Pour into a glass and drink as soon as possible. Serves 1.

Thyroid Tonic

Radishes are a traditional tonic for the thyroid gland.

5 carrots, scrubbed well, tops removed, ends trimmed
5-6 radishes
1 lemon, peeled
½ cucumber, peeled if not organic

Cut produce to fit your juicer's feed tube. Juice ingredients and stir. Pour into a glass and drink as soon as possible. Serves 1-2.

Triple C

4 stalks organic celery with leaves, as desired
4 carrots, scrubbed well, tops removed, ends trimmed
¼ small head green cabbage

Cut produce to fit your juicer's feed tube. Juice ingredients and stir. Pour into a glass and drink as soon as possible. Serves 1-2.

Tomato Florentine

2 tomatoes
4-5 sprigs basil
1 large handful of spinach
1 lemon, peeled

Juice one tomato. Wrap the basil in several spinach leaves. Turn off the machine and add the spinach and basil. Turn the machine back on and gently tap to juice them. Juice the remaining tomato and lemon. Stir juice, pour in a glass, and drink as soon as possible. Serves 1.

Veggie Time

4 carrots, scrubbed well, tops removed, ends trimmed
1 turnip, scrubbed well
1 lemon, peeled
2-inch chunk jicama, scrubbed or peeled if not organic
1 handful watercress
1 garlic clove

Cut produce to fit your juicer's feed tube. Juice ingredients and stir. Pour into a glass and drink as soon as possible. Serves 1-2.

Waldorf Twist

1 green apple
3 stalks organic celery with leaves
1 lemon, peeled

Cut produce to fit your juicer's feed tube. Juice ingredients and stir. Pour into a glass and drink as soon as possible. Serves 1.

Weight-Loss Buddy

Jerusalem artichoke juice combined with carrot and beet is a traditional remedy for satisfying cravings for sweets and junk food. The key is to sip it slowly when you get a craving for high-fat or high-carb foods.

3–4 carrots, scrubbed well, tops removed, ends trimmed
1 Jerusalem artichoke, scrubbed well
1 cucumber, peeled if not organic
1 lemon, peeled
½ small beet, scrubbed well, with stems and leaves

Cut produce to fit your juicer's feed tube. Juice ingredients and stir. Pour into a glass and drink as soon as possible. Serves 1.

Wheatgrass Light

1 green apple, washed
1 handful wheatgrass, rinsed
½ lemon, peeled
2-3 sprigs mint, rinsed (optional)

Cut produce to fit your juicer's feed tube. Start with apple and juice all ingredients and stir. Pour into a glass and drink as soon as possible. Serves 1.

SAVORY SMOOTHIES AND COLD SOUPS

These easy-to-make raw soups and savory smoothies are great for lunch or dinner. Some are even good for breakfast. Actually, you can take just about any juice recipe you like pour it in a blender, and add an avocado, and you have a raw soup.

Quick Energy Soup

> 1 cup fresh carrot juice (5-7 medium carrots, or
>   approximately 1 pound, yield about 1 cup)
> 1 lemon, peeled
> 1-inch chunk gingerroot
> 1 avocado, peeled and seed removed
> ½ tsp. ground cumin

Juice the carrots, lemon, and ginger. Pour the juice in a blender. Add the avocado and cumin and blend until smooth. Serve chilled. Serves 1.

Cherie's Awesome Green Smoothie

> 1 avocado, peeled, seeded, and cut in quarters
> 1 cup raw spinach
> ½ English cucumber, peeled and cut in chunks
> Juice of 1 lime
> 1 Tbsp. green powder of choice (optional)
> 2-3 Tbsp. ground almonds (optional)

Combine all ingredients in a blender and blend well until smooth. Sprinkle ground almonds on top, as desired. Serves 2.

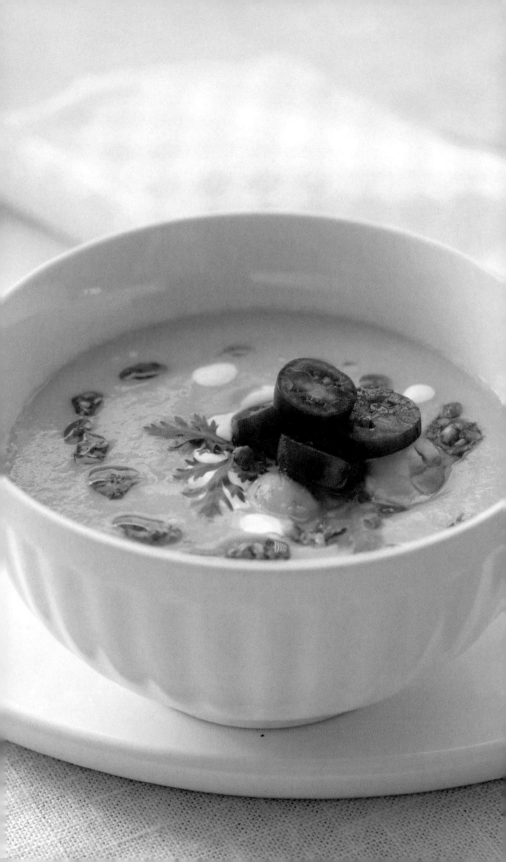

Icy Spicy Gazpacho

Chili peppers actually induce the brain to secrete endorphins, those brain chemicals that are credited with the "runner's high." Endorphins block pain sensations and induce a kind of euphoria. When you are feeling great, you're less likely to go on a food binge and pack on the pounds. Also, radishes are known to stimulate the thyroid, and an efficient thyroid is a key to weight loss and maintenance.

> 2 tomatoes, cut in chunks
> 1 cup fresh carrot juice (about 5-7 carrots)
> 1 lemon, juiced, peeled, if putting it through a juice
> machine
> 2 Tbsp. cilantro, rinsed and chopped
> ¼ tsp. Celtic sea salt
> ¼ tsp. ground cumin
> ¼ small jalapeño, chopped (more if you like it hot)
> 3 radishes

Place the tomato chunks in a freezer bag and freeze until solid. Pour the carrot and lemon juices into a blender and add the frozen tomato chunks, cilantro, salt, cumin, jalapeño, and radishes. Blend on high speed until smooth but slushy; serve immediately. Serves 2.

Minty Green Delight

> 1 avocado, peeled, seeded, and cut in quarters
> 1 cup raw spinach
> ½ English cucumber, peeled and cut in chunks
> ½–¾ cup coconut milk*
> Juice of 1 lime
> 1 Tbsp. green powder of choice (optional)
> 2-3 Tbsp. ground almonds (optional)

Combine all ingredients, except almonds, in a blender and blend well until smooth. Sprinkle ground almonds on top, as desired. Serves 2.

---

* The best coconut milk can be found in plastic pouches in the frozen section of Asian stores.

Cherie's Yummy Energy Soup

2-3 carrots, scrubbed
2-3 stalks celery with leaves, as desired
½ cucumber, peeled if not organic
½ lemon, peeled
Handful of parsley
1-2-inch chunk gingerroot, peeled
1 avocado, peeled and seeded
Garnish options: grated zucchini, chopped fresh corn, or
    crunchy sprouts such as pea, lentil, and bean

Juice the carrots, celery, cucumber, lemon, parsley, and gingerroot. Pour the juice in a blender and add the avocado. Blend until smooth. Pour into bowls and serve immediately. You may garnish with any of the optional additions for a crunchy topper. Serves 2.

Yummy Yam Bisque

1½ cups yam juice (about 2 large yams)
1 cup almond, oat, or rice milk
1 avocado, peeled and seeded
¼ cup red onion, chopped
1 tsp. nutmeg
¼ tsp. cinnamon
¼ tsp. ground allspice
¼ tsp. ground mace
¼ tsp. cardamom

Juice about two large yams to yield about 1½ cup of yam juice. Let the juice sit in a large measuring cup or bowl until the starch settles to the bottom. It will look thick and white. This should take about an hour. Pour off the clear juice, but not the starch, as this will make the soup gritty. Pour the yam juice and milk into a blender. Add the avocado and onion and blend until smooth. Add the spices and blend until smooth. Serves 2.

The Health Nut

To kill molds, add ½ tsp. ascorbic acid to the pineapple juice while nuts are soaking overnight.

> 1 cup unsweetened pineapple juice (juice one about quarter small pineapple, if making fresh juice)
> 10 almonds, whole or blanched
> 1 Tbsp. sunflower seeds
> 1 Tbsp. sesame seeds
> 1 Tbsp. flaxseed
> 1 Tbsp. chia seeds (optional)
> 1 cup chopped parsley
> ½ cup almond, rice, or oat milk
> ½ tsp. pure vanilla extract
> 1 Tbsp. protein powder
> 6 ice cubes

Place the pineapple juice, nuts, and seeds in a bowl. Cover and soak overnight. Place this nut and seed mixture with the juice in the blender and add the parsley, milk, vanilla, protein powder, and ice cubes. Blend on high speed until smooth. This smoothie will be a bit chewy because of the nuts and seeds. It makes a great breakfast. Serves 2–3.

Spinach-Avocado Soup

> 1 cucumber, peeled, cut in chunks
> 1 small jalapeño, seeded
> 1 avocado, peeled, seed removed
> Juice of 1 lemon
> 1–2 garlic cloves (optional)
> 1 Tbsp. cilantro
> 1 Tbsp. fresh parsley
> ¼ purple onion, finely chopped (for garnish)

Place all ingredients in a blender or food processor and purée until smooth. Pour into a bowl and add chopped onion, or any other chopped vegetables or herbs of choice as a garnish. Serves 2.

Creamy Tomato Soup

    1–2 tomatoes
    1 avocado, peeled, seed removed
    2 Tbsp. chopped sweet red bell pepper
    ¼ carrot, chopped in small pieces
    ½ cup rice, oat, or almond milk

Combine all ingredients in a blender and blend well. Pour into bowls. Serves 2.

Summer Corn Chowder

    2 cups fresh corn kernels cut off cob (about 2 large ears)
    1 cup almond, oat, or rice milk
    1 avocado, peeled, seed removed
    ¼ red bell pepper, cut in chunks
    2 tsp. finely minced red onion
    ½ tsp. ground cumin
    ½ tsp. Celtic sea salt
    Garnish: 1 Tbsp. each chopped parsley and minced red
        bell pepper (optional)

In a blender, combine the corn, milk, avocado, bell pepper, onion, cumin, and salt. Blend well. Pour into bowls and garnish with parsley and red pepper. Serves 2.

Refreshing Cucumber-Mint Soup

    1 cucumber, peeled if not organic and cut into chunks
    1 avocado, peeled, seed removed
    ¼–½ cup chopped fresh mint

Combine all ingredients in a blender and blend well. Pour into a bowl. Serves 1.

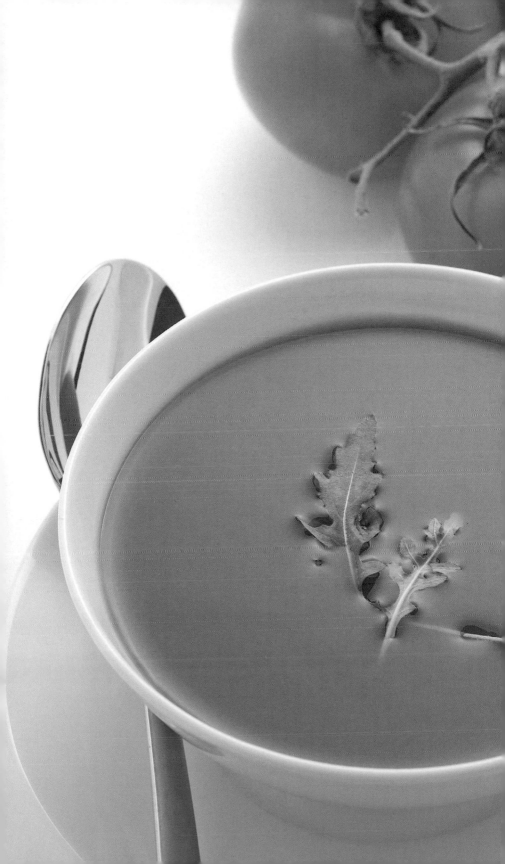

Skinny Shake

> 1 cucumber, peeled and cut in chunks
> 1 stalk celery, juiced or chopped into small pieces
> Juice of 1 lemon
> ½ tsp. freshly grated lemon peel

Place the cucumber chunks in a freezer bag and freeze them until solid. Combine the cucumber chunks in a blender with the celery, lemon juice, and lemon peel. Blend on high speed until well combined and slightly slushy. Serves 1.

Garden Tomato Soup

> 2 medium tomatoes
> 2 green onions (about 2 inches of tips and green), chopped
> ½ green bell pepper, chopped
> ½ cucumber, peeled if not organic
> 1 avocado, peeled, seed removed
> 1 tsp. Celtic sea salt
> Dash of hot sauce (optional)

Combine all ingredients in a blender and blend well. Pour into bowls. Serves 2.

French Tomato Basil Soup

> 3 medium tomatoes
> Juice of 1 lemon
> 1 avocado, peeled, seed removed
> 2 Tbsp. chopped fresh basil
> 1 small garlic clove
> Fresh basil leaves chopped for garnish (optional)

In a blender, blend the tomatoes until chunky. Add the lemon juice, avocado, basil, and garlic. Blend well. Pour into bowls and garnish with fresh basil leaves, as desired. Serves 2.

Kale Spinach Soup

> 3 large kale leaves
> 3 stalks celery
> 1 lemon, peeled
> 1 avocado, peeled, seed removed
> 1 cup spinach leaves

Juice the kale, celery, and lemon. Pour into a blender, add the avocado and spinach leaves, and blend well. Pour into bowls and serve. Serves 2.

Tomato Asparagus Soup

10 stalks asparagus, chopped
4 tomatoes, cut in chunks
3–4 sun-dried tomatoes
2 garlic cloves
¼ cup fresh parsley, chopped
¼ cup lemon juice
½ red bell pepper, chopped
1 tsp. Celtic sea salt
1 avocado, peeled, seed removed

Combine asparagus, tomatoes, sun-dried tomatoes, garlic, parsley, lemon juice, bell pepper, and salt in a blender and blend well. Add the avocado and blend well. Pour into bowls and serve. Serves 2.

Creamy Tomatillo Soup

1 cucumber, peeled and cut in chunks
2 tomatillos
1 lime (peeled and seeded), cut in chunks
2 cups fresh spinach
½ cup almond, oat, or rice milk
1 avocado, peeled, seed removed
4–6 ice cubes

Combine the cucumber, tomatillos, lime, spinach, and milk in a blender. Blend well. Add the avocado and ice cubes and blend again until smooth. Pour into bowls. Serves 2.

Refreshing Salsa Shake

2 cups tomatoes, cut in chunks
1 cup fresh cucumber juice
Juice of 1 lemon
½ tsp. freshly grated lemon peel, preferably organic
¼ daikon radish, chopped
Dash of cayenne pepper

Place tomato chunks in a freezer bag and freeze them until solid. Pour the cucumber juice and lemon juice in a blender and add the frozen tomato chunks, lemon peel, daikon radish, and cayenne pepper. Blend on high speed until smooth but slushy, and serve immediately. Serves 1–2.

Tomato Cooler

2 cups tomatoes, chopped
1 avocado, peeled, seed removed, cut in chunks
Juice of 1 lemon
½ cup almond, oat, or rice milk
½ tsp. freshly grated lemon peel, preferably organic
½ tsp. balsamic vinegar
Dash of cayenne pepper (optional)

Place the tomato chunks in a freezer bag and freeze until solid. Combine the tomato chunks, avocado, lemon juice, milk, lemon peel, balsamic vinegar, and cayenne pepper (as desired) in a blender. Blend on high speed until smooth but a bit slushy, and serve immediately. Serves 1–2.

Carrot Cooler

3 medium tomatoes, cut into chunks
1½ cups fresh carrot juice (about 5–6 large carrots)
2 Tbsp. fresh lemon juice
1 tsp. Celtic sea salt
1 garlic clove, peeled

Place the tomato chunks in a freezer bag and freeze until solid. Pour the carrot juice, lemon juice, and salt in a blender, and add the tomato chunks and garlic; blend on high speed until smooth but a bit slushy. Serve immediately. Serves 2.

Cucumber Dill Soup

1¼ cups fresh cucumber juice (about I large or 2
    medium cucumbers, peeled if not organic)
2 stalks celery with leaves, juiced
1 avocado, peeled, seed removed
1 garlic clove, peeled
½ cup almond, oat, or rice milk
½ cup parsley, coarsely chopped
2 tsp. red onion, chopped
3 tsp. fresh or 1–2 tsp. dried dill weed

Pour the cucumber and celery juices into a blender. Add the avocado, garlic, milk, parsley, onion, and dill. Blend on high speed until smooth and serve immediately. This soup is not good if it sits. Serves 2.

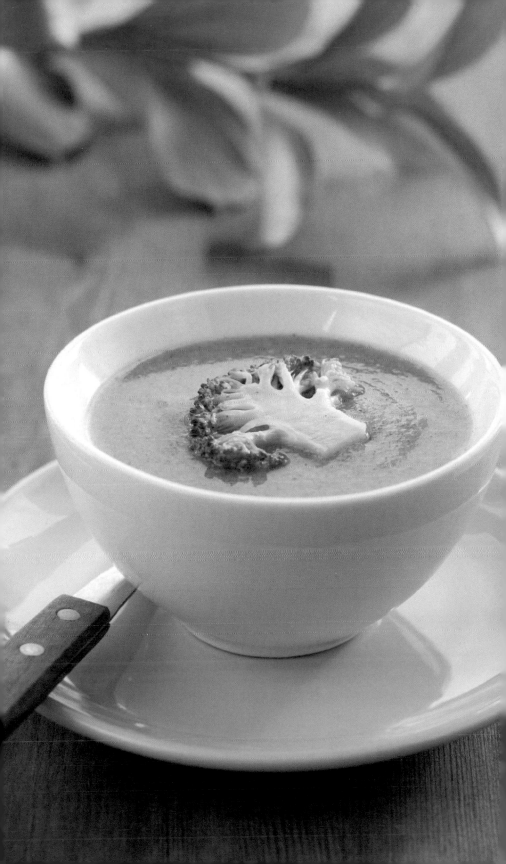

GENTLY WARMED SOUPS

If you keep the temperature at 105 degrees Fahrenheit, these soups will be considered raw food. This means you are preserving enzymes and vitamins so you can get the most nutrition from the food you are eating. If you don't have a thermometer, you can gauge the temperature by placing your finger in the soup to test when it is just warmed, not hot. That should be close to the right temperature.

Broccoli Soup

> 1 cup vegetable stock
> 1–2 cups broccoli, chopped
> ½ onion, chopped
> 1 red or yellow bell pepper, chopped
> 1–2 stalks celery, chopped
> 1 avocado, peeled and seeded
> 1 tsp. Celtic sea salt
> ½ tsp. cumin
> 1 tsp. of grated ginger (optional)
> Squeeze of lemon (optional)

Gently warm the vegetable stock, keeping the temperature at 105 degrees. Add the broccoli and onion and warm for 5 minutes. Turn off heat. Then add the bell pepper and celery for an additional 5 minutes. Pour the mixture in a blender and purée the broccoli, onion, bell pepper, and celery with the broth until smooth. Add the avocado and blend until smooth. Add the sea salt; then add cumin and blend. Pour soup in bowls. If using ginger, add to the top of the soup and stir in. A squeeze of lemon is nice; add as desired.

Vegetable Medley

> 2 cups water or vegetable broth
> 1 cup green beans, chopped
> 1 cup asparagus, chopped
> 2 carrots, chopped
> 2 stalks celery, chopped
> ½ onion, chopped
> 1 tsp. Celtic sea salt
> Pinch of mace (optional)

Pour water or vegetable broth into a soup pot. Add the vegetables and gently warm for about 10 minutes, or until vegetables are just slightly tender. Pour ingredients with the water or vegetable broth into a blender, add the mace, if using, and sea salt, and blend well. Pour into bowls. Serves 2.

Cream of Cauliflower Soup

½ onion chopped
3 stalks celery, chopped
1 head cauliflower, chopped
1 Tbsp. virgin coconut oil
1 cup almond or rice milk
½ tsp. sea salt
Pepper to taste (optional)

Lightly steam onion, celery, and cauliflower for about 5 minutes or until just tender. Combine in a blender with the coconut oil, milk, and salt. Blend well. Pour into bowls. Serves 2.

Creamy Red Pepper Soup

3 large red bell peppers
6 garlic cloves
1 cup almond, oat, or rice milk
1 Tbsp. balsamic vinegar
2 tsp. Celtic sea salt
6 fresh basil leaves, rinsed
Garnish: chopped fresh basil (optional)

Lightly steam the peppers and garlic for about 5 minutes or just until tender. Cut the peppers into chunks. Pour the milk into a blender and add the peppers, garlic, balsamic vinegar, salt, and basil. Blend on high speed until smooth. Pour into bowls and garnish with fresh basil, as desired. Serve immediately. Serves 1-2.

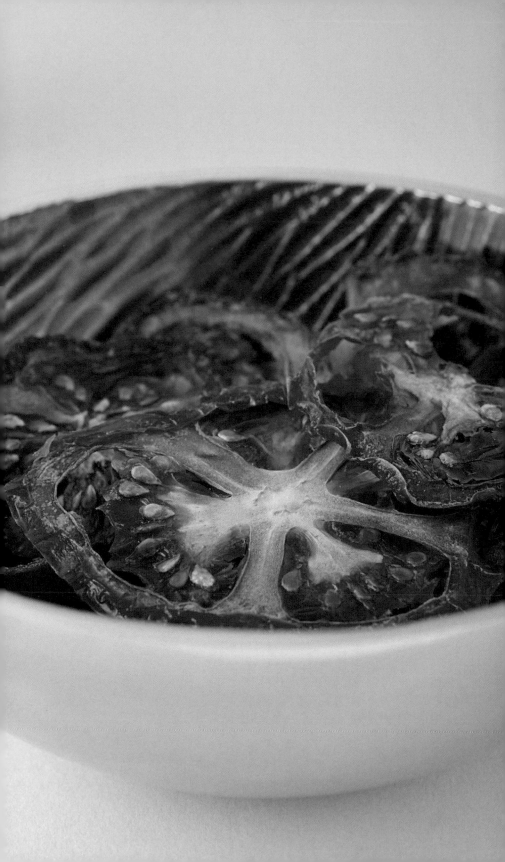

DEHYDRATED FOODS

Dehydrated foods make great snacks that can help you lose weight much more easily because they offer taste satisfaction without a lot of calories. For example, Kale Chips (page below) are very low in calories and exceptionally high in nutrients such as calcium, magnesium, and vitamin K. Onion Rings (page 196), Dehydrated Tomatoes and Basil, Garlicky Jicama Crackers (page 198), and Dehydrated Zucchini make wonderful snacks or accompaniment to meals and offer bursts of flavor along with fiber, enzymes, and a cornucopia of nutrients. It doesn't take much time to prepare them, and the rewards are great.

There are a number of schools of thought as to what the best temperature is to preserve the most enzymes and vitamins. If you want to get a dehydrator, see Appendix A.

Kale Chips

1 bunch kale
¼ cup apple cider or coconut vinegar
¼ cup fresh lemon juice
¼ cup extra-virgin olive oil
Pinch of cayenne pepper
½ tsp. Celtic sea salt
2 tsp. garlic, minced or pressed (optional)

Wash the kale and then cut it into 3-inch long strips and set aside to dry. Add vinegar, lemon juice, and olive oil to a blender and process until well combined. Then stir in the cayenne pepper, if using. Add the kale strips to the emulsion and massage the mixture into each leaf strip. Shake off excess marinade and place kale pieces on dehydrator sheets. Sprinkle with sea salt and garlic, if using, and dehydrate for about 7–8 hours at 105 degrees or until crisp. (Chips will get smaller as they dehydrate.)

These chips are so delicious I'll bet you won't have any left to store.

Onion Rings

3-5 onions (yellow, white, Walla Walla sweets)
¼ cup apple cider or coconut vinegar
¼ cup fresh lemon juice
¼ cup extra-virgin olive oil
½ tsp. Celtic sea salt
Pinch of cayenne pepper
2 tsp. garlic, minced or pressed (optional)

Cut onions into thin slices and set aside. Add vinegar, lemon juice, olive oil, and sea salt to a blender and process until well combined. Then stir in the cayenne pepper and minced garlic, if using. Add the onion slices to the emulsion and marinate for several hours. Shake off excess marinade so that onion rings are not dripping with marinade. Place onion rings on dehydrator sheets and dehydrate for about 7-8 hours at 105 degrees or until crisp.

Dehydrated Zucchini Chips

Slice zucchini into thin rounds and sprinkle with a little Celtic sea salt, as desired. You can also sprinkle your favorite seasoning on them. Place zucchini slices on dehydrator sheets and dehydrate for about 12 hours at 105 degrees or until crispy. They are surprisingly sweet and delicious. I actually like them best plain with nothing on them.

Dehydrated Tomatoes and Basil

Slice tomatoes thinly and put a fresh basil leaf on top of each slice, once you've placed them on a dehydrator sheet. Dehydrate for about 12 hours at 105 degrees or until crispy

Dehydrated Potato Chips

7 large, well scrubbed Yukon Gold (or other golden) potatoes, sliced (you may also use sweet potatoes or yams)
¼ cup extra-virgin olive oil or fresh lemon juice
¼ cup apple cider or coconut vinegar
Celtic sea salt to taste
Garlic powder to taste
Onion powder to taste
Dash of cayenne pepper (optional)

Slice the potatoes as thin as possible (paper thin works best; use a mandolin or spiral slicer for best results). Soak potato slices covered in cool water for several hours to get rid of some of the starch. Pat dry. Dip potato in marinade of fresh lemon juice or an emulsion of vinegar and olive oil to retard discoloration. Layer on dehydrator sheet. Sprinkle lightly with savory sprinkles (sea salt, garlic powder, onion powder, cayenne pepper) of choice. Dehydrate 8-10 hours at 105 degrees or until crispy and crunchy. Check frequently as the thinner potatoes will dry more quickly than thicker slices. Fills a 9-tray dehydrator.

Broccoli Latkes

1½ pounds of broccoli (you can use the stems)
½ pound of daikon radish
1 medium onion, cut into chunks
1 cup tahini
1 tsp. Celtic sea salt
½ tsp. black pepper

Place broccoli and daikon radish in the food processor and process until shredded. Scoop this mixture into a bowl. Add the chunks of onion to the food processor and process until in small pieces; add to the bowl. Blend together the tahini, salt, and pepper. Add this mixture to the vegetables in the bowl and mix well with your hands. Form into patties about 3 inches in diameter on dehydrator sheets. Dehydrate 8-10 hours and then turn them over carefully; dehydrate another 8-10 hours or until completely dry. Makes about 27 crackers.

Corn Crackers

½ cup golden flax seeds soaked in 2 cups purified water
   overnight
½ cup almonds soaked in 1 cup purified water
   overnight
2 cups fresh corn cut from the cob
3 Tbsp. chopped onion
1 tsp. cumin
2 tsp. Celtic sea salt

Blend all ingredients well in a food processor. Spread in rounds on a dehydrator sheet and dehydrate about 15 hours or until crisp. Makes about 36 crackers.

Garlicky Jicama Crackers

1 tomato, diced
1 red or yellow bell pepper, minced
1 tsp. Celtic sea salt
¼ cup extra-virgin olive oil
8-10 garlic cloves, minced or pressed
1 tsp. fresh oregano, finely chopped, or ½ tsp. dried
1 tsp. fresh basil, finely chopped, or ½ tsp. dried
1 medium jicama, thinly sliced

Combine all ingredients except the jicama in a bowl and mix well. Arrange jicama slices on a dehydrator sheet. Spoon about 1 tsp. of the tomato mixture onto each jicama slice and spread evenly. Dehydrate for about 24 hours at 105 degrees or until the jicama cracker is crisp. (Jicama will curl at edges.) Makes 12-15 crackers.

Veggie Crackers

1 onion, chopped
2 celery stalks, chopped
1 yellow or red bell pepper, chopped
1 tomato, chopped
1 large carrot, chopped
½ cup green peas
½ cup fresh corn cut from cob, or frozen
½ cup sesame seeds, soaked for several hours

Place all ingredients in a food processor and blend until almost smooth but slightly chunky. Drop a heaping teaspoon of batter at a time onto the dehydrator sheet, and swirl around with a spoon or pat with your fingers (dipped in a little water if they get sticky) to make cracker rounds. Dehydrate for about 8 hours and then flip the crackers. Dehydrate for another 6–10 hours at 105 degrees or until crispy. Makes about 15 crackers.

Seed Crackers

> 1 cup flaxseeds soaked in 2 cups purified water
>   overnight
> 1 cup sunflower seeds soaked overnight
> 1 cup almonds soaked overnight
> 1 cup yellow bell pepper, chopped
> 1 cup yellow squash, chopped
> ½ cup celery, chopped
> 3 Tbsp. fresh oregano or 1½ Tbsp. dried
> 1 Tbsp. onion powder
> 2 tsp. Celtic sea salt

Blend flaxseeds, sunflower seeds, and nuts in a food processor until smooth. Drop a heaping teaspoon of batter at a time onto the dehydrator sheet, and swirl around with a spoon or pat with your fingers (dipped in a little water if they get sticky) to make cracker rounds. Dehydrate for about 8 hours and then flip the crackers. Dehydrate for another 6–10 hours at 105 degrees or until crispy. Makes about 36 crackers.

Guilt-free "Bacon"

> ¼ cup extra-virgin olive oil
> 4 Tbsp. apple cider vinegar
> 2 Tbsp. honey
> 1 tsp. ground black pepper
> 1 eggplant, thinly sliced into strips

Mix together the olive oil, vinegar, honey, and pepper, and marinate the eggplant strips for at least 2 hours in the mixture. Then place the strips on a dehydrator sheet and dehydrate for 12 hours at 105 degrees. Turn strips over and dehydrate another 12 hours.

BREAKFAST RECIPES

Sprouted Buckwheat Groats

For your morning cereal, sprouted buckwheat is great served with rice, oat, or almond milk, some ground almonds, and cinnamon.

Put 1 cup (or as much as you want) of raw buckwheat groat seeds into a bowl or your sprouter. Add 2-3 times as much cool, purified water. Swish seeds around to assure even water contact for all. Allow seeds to soak overnight. Drain off the soak water. Rinse thoroughly with cool water. Groats create very starchy water; it's very thick! They won't sprout well unless rinsed well, so rinse until the water runs clear. Drain thoroughly. You can add to your sprouter at this time or simply put the sprouts in a colander and cover with a tea towel. Set out of direct sunlight at room temperature (70 degrees is optimal; if it's too cold they won't sprout). Rinse and drain again in 4-8 hours. Yields approximately 1½ cups of sprouts.

Sprouted Rye Cereal

Rye harvested immature or handled improperly can have a strong, unpleasant flavor. If it molds, discard (ergot mold is possible).

Soak rye seeds 8-14 hours, and sprout 1-1½ days. Use a sprouter or colander as in the Sprouted Buckwheat Groats (above). Rye is a nice sprout with good flavor.

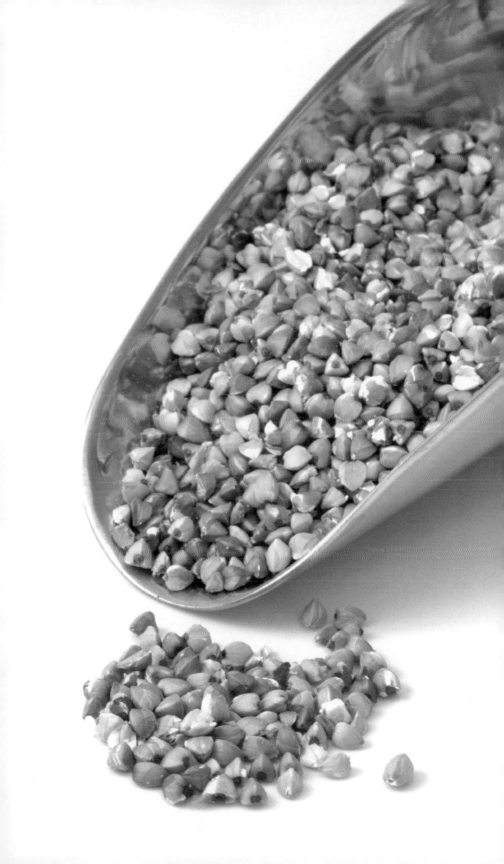

SALAD DRESSINGS

Citrus-Balsamic Vinaigrette

Orange juice combines nicely with balsamic vinegar to make a delicious variation to the basic balsamic vinaigrette.

2 Tbsp. balsamic vinegar
½ tsp. Celtic sea salt, or to taste
¼ tsp. freshly ground black pepper, or to taste
3 Tbsp. orange juice (fresh is best)
1 Tbsp. Dijon mustard
1 large garlic clove, pressed
½ cup extra-virgin olive oil

Combine all ingredients except the oil and mix well. While whisking, drizzle in oil very slowly in a steady stream until an emulsion is formed. Makes 1 cup (about 16 servings).

Lemon-Tarragon Vinaigrette

¼ cup fresh lemon juice
½ tsp. lemon zest
½ tsp. Celtic sea salt, or to taste
¼ tsp. freshly ground black pepper, or to taste
1 large garlic clove, pressed
¾ cup extra-virgin olive oil
2 Tbsp. fresh tarragon or 1 Tbsp. dried

Combine all ingredients except the oil and tarragon and mix well. While whisking, drizzle in oil very slowly in a steady stream until an emulsion is formed. Add tarragon and mix well. Makes 1 cup (about 16 servings).

Lemon Vinaigrette

Follow the recipe instructions for Lemon-Tarragon Vinaigrette (above) and omit the tarragon.

Main Course Raw Vegan

Asian Salad

2 zucchini, sliced into strips with a vegetable peeler or
    mandolin
2 large handfuls of bean sprouts, approximately 2 cups
¾ cup chopped almonds or cashews
1 red or yellow bell pepper, sliced into strips
4 green onions, diced
½ cup fresh cilantro, chopped
Juice from one lime
1 Tbsp. extra-virgin olive oil
½ tsp. Celtic sea salt

Toss all ingredients together in a bowl until well coated. Serves
2–3.

Sunshine "Eggless" Salad or Sunshine "Eggless" Salad Roll-ups

½ cup pure water
½ cup fresh lemon juice
1½ tsp. turmeric
1 tsp. Celtic sea salt, adjust to taste
1½ cups raw macadamia nuts or cashews (sweeter with
    cashews)
½ cup green onion, diced
½ cup celery, diced
⅓ cup red bell pepper, diced (optional)

Place all ingredients (except diced green onion, celery, and
red bell pepper) into a food processor, fitted with an S blade.
Process until very smooth. Transfer to a bowl and stir in the
green onion, celery, and red bell pepper. Mix well.

Serve as a dip with veggies or place onto romaine lettuce
leaves for a quick and easy wrap. May be served as an
appetizer also. Cut cucumber slices diagonally and lay out
onto service platter. Place 1 Tbsp. of Sunshine "Eggless" Salad
onto each cucumber slice. Garnish with sprigs of fresh parsley
or sliced green onion. Serves 16–20 appetizer size; 8–10 as
roll-up sandwich.

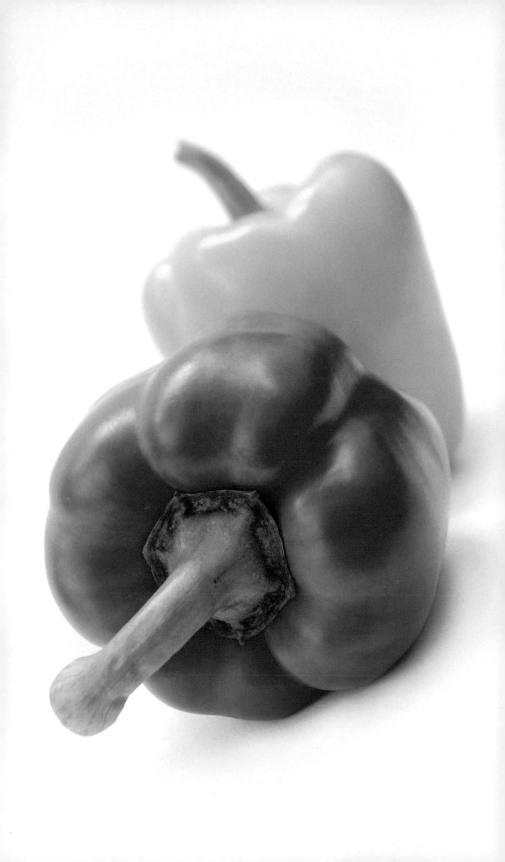

South of the Border Lettuce Wraps

2 ripe avocados
3 tomatoes, diced
½ jalapeño pepper, diced
2 Tbsp. yellow onion, diced
3 fresh garlic cloves, minced
¼ cup fresh cilantro, chopped
Kernels cut from one ear raw corn
2 tsp. fresh lime juice
6–8 large lettuce leaves

In a medium sized bowl, mash the avocados. Add the remaining ingredients and stir until well mixed Spread 2-3 Tbsp. of this mixture onto lettuce leaves and wrap. Serves 6–8.

Stuffed Bell Peppers

6 medium carrots, chopped
1–2 celery stalks, chopped
1 large or 2 small ripe avocados
1 tsp. dulse or Celtic sea salt
½ cup chopped cucumber
½ cup chopped tomato
½ tsp. cumin
1 large red or yellow bell pepper
Raw sunflower seeds for garnish

Place carrots and celery in a food processor and process until pulp consistency or use carrot and celery pulp leftover from juicing. Transfer the pulp to a bowl. Remove the flesh from the avocado(s) and, using a fork, mash the avocado into the carrot-celery pulp. Add the dulse or salt, cucumber, tomato, and cumin, and mix well. Cut bell pepper in half; scoop out the seeds and stuff with the carrot-avocado mixture. Top each stuffed pepper with 1 tsp. of sunflower seeds. Serves 2.

Jalapeño Nut Burgers

> 1 cup walnuts, soaked for 4 hours
> ¼ cup sun-dried tomatoes, soaked until very soft; reserve
>   ⅛ cup soaking water
> 1 jalapeño pepper, finely chopped
> ½ onion, finely chopped
> 1 tsp. hamburger seasoning
> 1 tsp. Celtic sea salt
> ½ tsp. black pepper

In a food processor, combine walnuts, sun-dried tomatoes and soaking water until you achieve a meat consistency. Remove from processor. Place the nut mixture in a bowl, and combine with the jalapeño peppers, onions, seasoning, salt, and pepper. Shape into 6 patties. Dehydrate at 105 degrees for 3–4 hours. Serves 6.

Spicy Peanut Sauce Over Zucchini Noodles

This sauce tastes fantastic, and if you let it sit a bit, it gets even better.

> ½ cup raw peanut butter or almond butter
> 1–2 tsp. hot chili oil
> 2–3 tsp. tamari, Nama Shoyu, or organic soy sauce
> 1 garlic clove, minced
> 1 tsp. virgin coconut oil
> 2–3 yellow summer squash or zucchini, made into
>   noodles with a spiral or spirooli slicer

In a food processor combine everything except the coconut oil and squash noodles until well blended. (Adjust tamari, shoyu or soy sauce, and chili oil to taste.) Add the oil just until the sauce is of the consistency you like.

Serve over summer squash or zucchini noodles. Yellow summer squash is a bit sturdier than zucchini and works well with the spicy peanut sauce. Serves 4.

Easy Phad Thai

3 zucchini, made into noodles with a spiral or spirooli slicer
1 package (3½ oz.) enoki mushrooms, trimmed and separated
3 green onions, thinly sliced
1 red bell pepper, cut into thin strips
10 snow peas
½ pound mung bean sprouts
½ lime, juiced
½ tsp. Celtic sea salt
1 Tbsp. extra-virgin olive oil

In a bowl, combine all the ingredients and stir well. Spoon Phad Thai Sauce over top and sprinkle topping over sauce. Serves 6.

Phad Thai Sauce

1 Tbsp. hiziki seaweed, soaked for 30 minutes or more in enough water to cover (optional)
½ cup raw almond butter
½ cup sun-dried tomatoes, soaked 2 hours
1 lime, chopped (including peel if organic)
4 garlic cloves, peeled and finely chopped or pressed
7 dates, pitted and chopped
½ cup extra-virgin olive oil
2 small Thai chilies or 1 jalapeño (do not remove seeds if you like it hot)
1½ Tbsp. fresh ginger, grated
1-2 Tbsp. tamari, plus extra if desired, or 1 tsp. Celtic sea salt
½ cup purified water
1 cup cilantro, loosely packed, chopped
Juice of ½ lemon or line (about 1½ Tbsp.)
1 Tbsp. maple syrup or date paste

Blend the hiziki, if using, almond butter, sun-dried tomatoes, lime, garlic, dates, olive oil, chilies, ginger, and tamari or sea salt with ½ cup water until creamy. Add additional ingredients and blend again.

Topping

1 cup almonds, chopped
½ cup cilantro, chopped
Handful bean sprouts

Raw Enchiladas

Corn Tortillas

5 ears of corn with kernels cut off the cob
2 Tbsp. psyllium husk (not seed)
Water as needed

To make the tortillas: Place the ingredients in a food processor and blend until smooth. Batter should be about the consistency of pancake batter. Place large spoonfuls of batter on dehydrator sheets. Using a spoon, swirl batter in a circular motion to shape into rounds to your desired tortilla size. Dehydrate about 4 hours. Flip tortillas and dehydrate another 2 hours or until no longer wet yet soft and easy to roll. Don't leave in the dehydrator too long, or the tortillas will get hard. If that happens, you can make tostadas. This recipe makes about 16 to 20 tortillas.

Filling

Raw corn kernels cut from 1 ear of corn
½ red bell pepper, chopped
½ onion, finely chopped
½ cup cilantro, chopped
½ zucchini, chopped

In a bowl, combine all ingredients and mix well.

To assemble enchiladas: Arrange tortillas on counter or breadboard. Top each tortilla with about 1 Tbsp. of filling. Place 1 Tbsp. of Nutty Cheese Sauce (page 212) or guacamole on top of the filling and roll each tortilla into an enchilada-style roll. It can be served with salsa. Serves 6–8.

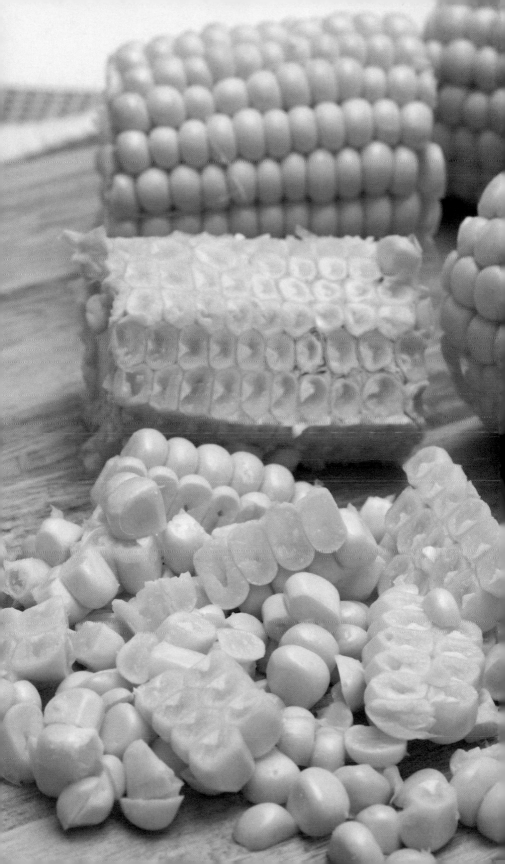

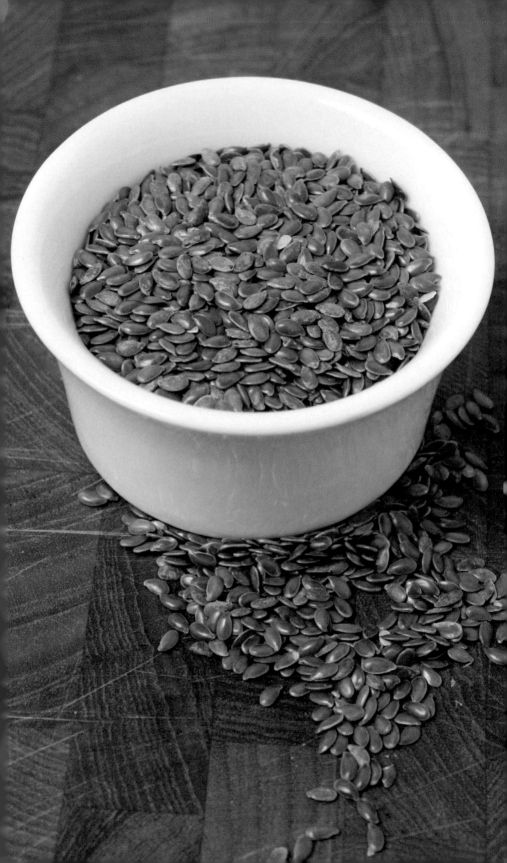

Gourmet Raw Pizza

This is a higher calorie recipe that should be enjoyed after you've reached your weight loss goal.

Raw Buckwheat Groat Pizza Dough (Crackers)

This recipe also makes a delicious Italian Buckwheat cracker.

2 cups sprouted buckwheat groats *
1-2 garlic cloves, chopped
¾ cup finely grated carrots (or use carrot pulp)
¾ cup soaked flaxseeds (soak overnight; they'll expand
    to about 1½ cups or use ground flaxseeds and extra
    water)
½ cup extra-virgin olive oil
1 Tbsp. Italian seasonings (or fresh herbs to taste)
1-2 tsp. Celtic sea salt
Water as needed (usually ½-1 cup)

Mix all ingredients together in a food processor. Start with buckwheat groats and garlic, followed by the rest of the ingredients. Coat a dehydrator sheet with a small amount of olive oil and scoop batches of dough (about a heaping tablespoon each) onto dehydrator sheets and swirl each scoop with a spoon to make rounds. You can make large pizza dough (about 6 inches in diameter), or you can make smaller individual rounds (about 3 inches in diameter). The smaller rounds are easier to serve and eat. Press out the dough evenly to about ⅛- to ¼-inch thick by patting the top with your fingertips or swirling with a spoon. If it gets too sticky, dip your fingers into some water to which you add a little olive oil. Once crust is pressed out evenly, dehydrate at 105 degrees for about 7 hours. Flip the crackers and dry another 7-10 hours or until crust is completely dry and crisp. (It should be crunchy for the best-tasting cracker.) To speed the drying process, you can transfer to the mesh rack for a couple of hours after you flip the crackers. Use a spatula when lifting dough, and be careful when transferring it not to break the crackers. Serves 16 (2 each).

NOTE: If crust is very dry and stored in a cool dry, airtight container, it can be kept fresh for several months.

---

* To sprout buckwheat, soak 1 cup raw buckwheat groats overnight; it will expand to about 2 cups. Drain and rinse well. Place on counter in a colander covered with a lightweight dish towel or in a sprouter for one day. Rinse several times while sprouting. (If you don't have time to sprout, you can use buckwheat that has been soaked at least 4 hours.

Nutty Cheese Sauce for Pizza Topping

1 cup macadamia nuts and 1 cup raw pine nuts,
    soaked, or 2 cups cashews, soaked (cashews are a
    bit sweeter and usually less expensive)
½ cup lemon juice
1½ tsp. Celtic sea salt
1 Tbsp. garlic, chopped
½ tsp. peppercorns, ground
Water as needed

Soak nuts first for several hours. Blend all ingredients until very creamy, about 3–4 minutes for the creamiest sauce. Add water as needed. This sauce will keep 3 days in the refrigerator in a covered container.

Yummy Marinara Sauce

This sauce is also great on raw spaghetti.

½ cup dried (or fresh) pineapple, soaked
2 cups chopped tomatoes
1 tsp. ginger, minced
2 Tbsp. garlic, minced
1 tsp. jalapeño, minced
⅓ cup fresh basil leaves, chopped and packed, or
    2 Tbsp. dried
¼ cup red bell pepper, chopped
⅓ cup sun-dried tomatoes, soaked
⅓ cup fresh oregano leaves, de-stemmed and
    chopped, or 2 Tbsp. dried
¼ cup Nama Shoyu or 1½ tsp. Celtic sea salt
1 cup extra-virgin olive oil

Blend all ingredients together in a food processor. If the sauce sets in the refrigerator for at least an hour, it will thicken and become more flavorful

To assemble pizza: Arrange Buckwheat Groat Pizza Dough crackers on a plate. Spoon about 2 tsp. of the Yummy Marinara Sauce on the top of each cracker. It should be thick and not run over the edges. Top with several little dollops of Nutty Cheese Sauce by placing about ½ tsp. of cheese sauce in a few places on top of the marinara sauce. If the Nutty Cheese Sauce is too thick, add a little water. It should still be thick and not at all runny. For a garnish, top pizza with finely chopped scallions, onions, black olives, or leeks.

Main Course Cooked Vegan Recipes

Springtime Vegetables With Cashew-Carrot Sauce

8–11 carrots, juiced
½ cup raw cashews
2 Tbsp. white or yellow miso
1 pound fresh asparagus
½ cup frozen peas
2 scallions or green onions, chopped
¼ cup marinated sun-dried tomatoes, thinly sliced
3 Tbsp. fresh basil, finely chopped
2 garlic cloves, pressed

Juice the carrots and reserve the juice. You should have 1½ cups carrot juice. In a blender or food processor, combine the juice, cashews, and miso; blend on high until the cashews are not gritty and the mixture is smooth and creamy.

Snap off the bottoms of the asparagus; cut the tender part into 1-inch chunks.

In a medium-size saucepan or skillet, combine the cashew-carrot juice mixture with the asparagus, peas, sun-dried tomatoes, basil, and garlic. Bring the sauce to a boil. Cover the pan and reduce the heat; simmer, stirring occasionally, for 4–5 minutes. Turn off the heat and let stand with the lid on. Spoon vegetable mixture over wild rice. Serves 6–8.

Moroccan Stew

2 Tbsp. virgin coconut oil
1½ cups onions, chopped
4 cups green cabbage, chopped
2 cups Jerusalem artichokes (sun chokes), chopped
1½ cups celery, chopped
1½ cups sliced carrots
1½ tsp. cumin
3 bay leaves
1 cup tomato sauce
1 cup purified water
2 cups cooked garbanzo beans (chickpeas)
2 tsp. Celtic sea salt
½ tsp. red pepper flakes
1 tsp. ground cumin
½ tsp. ground ginger
½ tsp. turmeric
½ tsp. cinnamon

In a large skillet, heat the oil over low heat. Add the onions and sauté until translucent. Add the cabbage, Jerusalem artichoke, celery, carrots, cumin, and bay leaves, and continue to sauté, stirring occasionally, for about 5 minutes. Add tomato sauce and water to a soup pot along with the sautéed vegetable mixture. Add the garbanzo beans, salt, pepper flakes, and spices. Cover and simmer about 45 minutes or until the vegetables are tender. Serves 6–8.

Chipotle Bean Soup

1 Tbsp. virgin coconut oil
1 onion, chopped
1½ cups dried navy, lima, or pinto beans
2 garlic cloves, chopped
2 chipotle chilies, soaked 10 minutes in cold water*
4 cups water or stock
2 tsp. Celtic sea salt
2 tsp. brown rice vinegar
Freshly ground pepper to taste

Soak beans overnight.
    Heat oil in a large soup pot and cook onion over medium heat until soft. Drain beans and add to onions along with garlic, chilies, and water. Bring heat to high until mixture starts to simmer. Reduce heat to low and cook for 1 hour, or until beans are soft. Remove chilies. For thicker, creamier soup, purée half the soup in a blender and then return it to the soup pot and mix well. Add the salt, vinegar, and pepper. Serves 6.

---

* Chipotle chilies add a smoked flavor that is similar to cooking beans with ham.

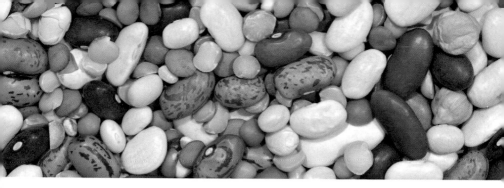

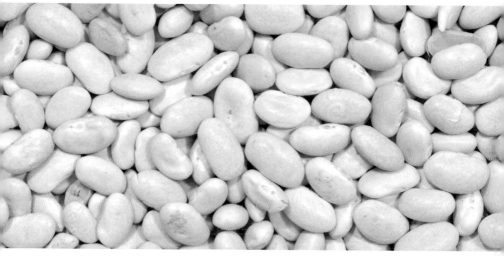

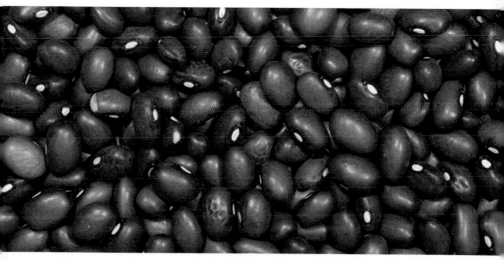

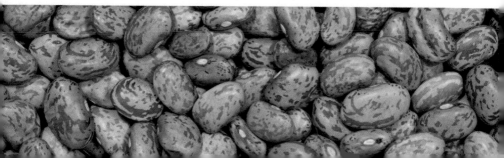

Red Lentil and Spinach Soup

1 Tbsp. virgin coconut oil
1 cup diced onion
1 cup diced leeks
2-3 garlic cloves, minced or pressed
1 cup dry red lentils
7 cups purified water
1 can (6 ounces) tomato paste
1 vegetable bouillon cube
1 large tomato, chopped
1 Tbsp. fresh lemon juice
4 cups spinach, chopped
Celtic sea salt and pepper to taste

Heat the oil in a small skillet on low heat. Add the onions, leeks, and garlic and sauté until onion is translucent. Place the lentils in a fine-mesh wire strainer and rinse well. In a soup kettle, combine lentils and water. Bring the water to a boil, then skim off any foam that forms on the top of the lentils. Add the tomato paste, bouillon cube, sautéed onions, leeks, and garlic. Reduce the heat and simmer for about 15 minutes. Add the chopped tomato, lemon juice, and chopped spinach along with the salt and pepper. Simmer for an additional 20 to 30 minutes or until lentils are tender. Serves 6.

Cashew Mushroom Loaf

1 Tbsp. virgin coconut oil
1 small onion, chopped
2 garlic cloves, pressed
12 oz. raw cashews
3 medium parsnips, cooked and mashed
1 tsp. dried rosemary
1 tsp. dried thyme
1 tsp. Celtic sea salt
1 Tbsp. virgin coconut oil
12 oz. fresh button mushrooms, chopped

Preheat oven to 350 degrees. Heat oil in a small skillet and sauté onion and garlic until onion is translucent. Grind the cashews and mix with the mashed parsnips, herbs, and salt. Add oil to the skillet again and sauté the chopped mushrooms until soft. Grease loaf pan with oil and press in half the nut mixture. Add the mushrooms, then top with the rest of the nut mixture. Press in well. Bake for 1 hour. Let stand for 10 minutes and remove from the pan. Slice to serve. Serves 6.

Cashew Vegetable Curry

1 medium eggplant, cut into 1-inch cubes (zucchini or
  summer squash can be substituted)
Celtic sea salt to taste
2 Tbsp. virgin coconut oil
1 onion, coarsely chopped
1 Tbsp. fresh ginger, grated
1 Tbsp. ground cumin
3 tsp. ground coriander
1 tsp. ground cinnamon
1 tsp. turmeric
¼ tsp. cayenne pepper
⅛ tsp. cardamom (optional)
1 cup purified water
½ cup coconut milk
1 medium yellow or red bell pepper, cut into 1-inch pieces
1 bunch spinach (about 10 ounces), stemmed, chopped
1 Tbsp. fresh lemon juice
¾ cup cashews

Put the eggplant cubes in a colander, sprinkle with a little sea salt, and let sit for 30 minutes. Heat the oil in a large saucepan over medium-high heat and sauté onion until translucent. Reduce the heat to medium-low and add the spices and cook for 5 minutes. Rinse the eggplant and add it to the onion mixture. Stir in the water and coconut milk. Cover and simmer on low for 15 minutes or until eggplant is tender. Add the bell pepper and cook 5 minutes. Add the spinach and lemon juice. Add salt as desired. Stir in cashews. Serve over wild or brown rice. Serves 4–6.

Broccoli-Ginger Stir-Fry

1 Tbsp. virgin coconut oil
4 Tbsp. minced fresh ginger
4 garlic cloves, minced
¼ onion, sliced into crescents
2 carrots, sliced
1 cup sliced mushrooms
1½ cup broccoli florets
2 cups boy choy or napa cabbage, chopped
1 small red or yellow bell pepper, cut into strips
½ cup red cabbage, chopped

Sauce

¼ cup tamari
2 Tbsp. brown rice vinegar
1 Tbsp. toasted sesame oil
Stevia to taste
3 Tbsp. sesame seeds

Heat the oil in a large skillet over medium-high heat. Add the ginger and garlic and cook for 2 to 3 minutes. Add the onion and carrots and cook for 2 minutes. Reduce the heat to medium and add the mushrooms and cook for 3 minutes or until onion is translucent. Add the broccoli and cook 2 to 3 minutes. Then add the boy choy, bell pepper, and red cabbage and cook for 2 minutes.

To make the sauce, in a small bowl combine the tamari, brown rice vinegar, sesame oil, and stevia. Add the sauce to the vegetable mixture in the skillet and cook for about 5 minutes over medium heat. Sprinkle with sesame seeds before serving. Serves 4.

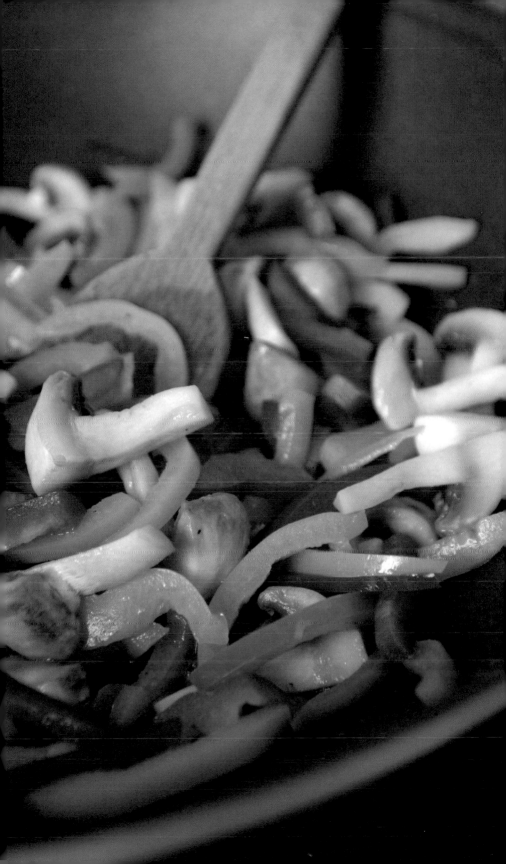

MAIN COURSE MEALS WITH FISH AND CHICKEN

Moroccan Chicken With Lemon and Olives

2 tsp. paprika
1 tsp. ground cumin
1 tsp. ground ginger
1 tsp. turmeric
½ tsp. cinnamon
¼ tsp. ground pepper
1 pastured or free-range chicken, cut into 8 pieces (or
    you can use just chicken thighs and legs)
2 Tbsp. virgin coconut oil
Celtic sea salt to taste
3 garlic cloves, minced
1 onion, chopped
1 Tbsp. lemon zest
½ cup purified water
1 cup pitted green olives
¼ cup fresh cilantro
¼ cup parsley

Combine all the spices in a large bowl. Rinse the chicken
and pat dry. Place it in the bowl, coating well with the spice
mixture. Let the chicken sit for one hour in the spices. In a large
heavy skillet, heat the oil on medium heat. Add the chicken
pieces, sprinkle lightly with salt, and brown skin side down for
5 minutes. Lower the heat to medium-low, add the garlic and
onions. Cover and let cook for 15 minutes. Add the lemon
zest, water, and green olives. Continue cooking another 45
minutes covered or until completely done. Spread cilantro
and parsley over top and serve. Serves 4–6.

Chicken Curry

1 Tbsp. virgin coconut oil
1 Tbsp. red or green curry paste
1 pound boneless, skinless chicken breasts, flattened
    and cut into bite-size pieces
1½ cups chicken stock
1 cup bamboo shoots, sliced
½ cup carrots, sliced
2 Tbsp. Thai fish sauce
Stevia to taste
½ cup fresh basil, chopped
½ cup cilantro, chopped

Heat the oil in a large skillet over low heat and sauté curry paste for about 2 minutes. Add the chicken and stir. Add the chicken stock and increase the heat to high. Stir until chicken is well coated with curry paste and chicken is opaque. Add the bamboo shoots and carrots. Cook for 2 minutes or until sauce comes to a boil. Add the fish sauce and stevia to taste. Lower the heat to medium, add the basil and cilantro and cook for 2 minutes. For a more flavorful dish, transfer to saucepan and cook on low heat for 15 to 20 minutes. Serves 4.

Garlic Dijon Halibut

1-1½ lb. halibut, cut into 4 pieces
¼ cup lemon juice
Celtic sea salt and pepper to taste

Topping

2 Tbsp. mayonnaise
2 Tbsp. green onions, chopped
2 tsp. fresh lemon juice
2 garlic cloves, pressed or minced
1 tsp. Dijon mustard
¼ tsp. hot sauce or pinch of cayenne pepper

On each side of the halibut, make 3 diagonal cuts 2 inches long and ½ inch deep. Place the halibut in a large shallow dish and pour the lemon juice over it. Marinate for 30 minutes at room temperature. Preheat the oven to 450 degrees F. Place the fish on a broiling pan and sprinkle with lemon juice from the marinade. Bake the fish for 15 minutes, or until it is opaque in the center. While the fish is baking, combine the mayonnaise, green onions, lemon juice, garlic, mustard, and hot sauce or cayenne. Mix well. Remove fish from oven when done. Turn the oven to broil. Sprinkle fish with salt and pepper. Spread the topping over the fish and broil for 2 minutes, or until the topping is golden brown. Serves 4.

Baked Tomato Snapper

4 snapper fillets, about 4 to 6 oz. each
1 medium onion, chopped
½ cup red or yellow bell pepper, chopped
½ cup sliced mushrooms
1 tsp. dried oregano
1 tsp. dried basil
½ tsp. dried tarragon
½ tsp. dried rosemary
1 16-oz. can stewed tomatoes
Celtic sea salt and pepper to taste

Preheat oven to 375 degrees. Place the fish in a baking dish and cover with the chopped vegetables. Sprinkle the herbs over the vegetables and top with the stewed tomatoes. Bake the fish for 30 to 40 minutes or until it is opaque inside and the sauce thickens a bit. Sprinkle with salt and pepper as desired before serving. Serves 4.

Turbo Diet Resource Guide

S IGN UP FOR Cherie's free Juice Newsletter at www.juiceladyinfo
.com.

Cherie's Web sites

- www.juiceladyinfo.com—information on juicing and weight loss
- www.cheriecalbom.com—information about Cherie's Web sites
- www.sleepawaythepounds.com—information about the Sleep Away the Pounds program and products
- www.gococonuts.com—information about the Coconut Diet and coconut oil
- www.ultimatesmoothie.com—information about *The Ultimate Smoothie Book* and healthy smoothies

Other books by Cherie and John Calbom

These books can be ordered at any of the Web sites above or by calling 866.843.8935.

- Cherie Calbom, *The Juice Lady's Guide to Juicing for Health* (Penguin)
- Cherie Calbom with John Calbom, *Juicing, Fasting, and Detoxing for Life* (Grand Central Wellness)
- Cherie Calbom and John Calbom, *Sleep Away the Pounds* (Warner Wellness)
- Cherie Calbom. *The Wrinkle Cleanse* (Avery)
- Cherie Calbom and John Calbom, *The Coconut Diet* (Warner)

- Cherie Calbom, John Calbom, and Michael Mahaffey,
  The Complete Cancer Cleanse (Warner)
- Cherie Calbom, *The Ultimate Smoothie Book* (Warner)

Juicers

Find out the best juicers recommended by Cherie Calbom. Call 866-8GETWEL (866.843.8935) or visit www.juiceladyinfo.com.

Dehydrators

Find out the best dehydrators recommended by Cherie Calbom. Call 866-8GETWEL (866.843.8935) or visit www.juiceladyinfo.com.

Lymphasizer

To view the Swing Machine (lymphasizer), visit www.juiceladyinfo .com or call 866-8GETWEL (866.843.8935).

Powders

To purchase or get information on Barley Max, Carrot Max, and Beet Max powders, call 866.843.8935. (These powders are ideal for when you travel or when you can't get juice.)

Virgin coconut oil

For more information on virgin coconut oil, go to www.gococonuts .com or call 866.843.8935. To save money, order larger sizes such as gallons or quarts, which you won't typically find in the stores.

Supplements

- Multivitamins by Thorne Research: call 866.843.8935
- Digestive enzymes Ness Formula #4 and #16 are excellent to aid digestion. Taken between meals, they help clean up undigested proteins. With the addition of enzymes, you should notice that your hair and nails grow better. Call 866-8GETWEL (866.843.8935).
- Calcium Citrate or Calcium Citramate (contains both calcium citrate-malate and malic acid; offers good solubility and superb absorption when compared to other forms of calcium) by Thorne Research: call 866.843.8935

- Magnesium Citrate or Magnesium Citramate (as Magnesium Citrate-Malate and malic acid) by Thorne Research: call 866.843.8935
- Vitamin C with bioflavonoids or Buffered C Powder (contains ascorbic acid, calcium, magnesium, and potassium) by Thorne Research or Allergy Research: call 866.843.8935
- Vitamin D$_3$ (1,000 or 5000 mg) by Thorne Research: call 866.843.8935

Colon cleanse products

Call 866.843.8935 for more information on Cherie's fiber recommendations below.

- Medibulk by Thorne (psyllium powder, prune powder, apple pectin)
- Blessed Herbs Colon Cleanse in Peppermint or Ginger

Liver/gallbladder cleanse products

- S.A.T. by Thorne (milk thistle, artichoke, turmeric) along with Cysteplus (N-Acetyl-L-Cysteine) and Lipotropein (vitamins, minerals, L-Methionine, and herbs including dandelion, beet leaf, and black radish root)— call 866.843.8935
- Chinese herbal tinctures (4-part kit) to use with Cherie's Liver Detox Program—call 866.843.8935

***Candida albicans* cleanse products**

- Blessed Herbs Total Body Cleanse—visit www.juice ladyinfo.com or call 866.843.8935

Parasite cleanse products

- Blessed Herbs Total Body Cleanse—visit www.juice ladyinfo.com or call 866.843.8935
- Worm Squirm I and II; Arise & Shine—call 866.843.8935
- Silver Creek Labs ParaCease & ParaAssist—call 800.493.1146

Kidney cleanse herbs

- Arise & Shine Kidney Life—call 888.557.4463
- Dr. Schultz's Kidney Cleanse Detox Kit

Heavy metal and toxic compounds cleanse products
For all these products, call 866.843.8935.

- Captomer by Thorne (Succinic acid from 100 mg DMSA)—chelates heavy metals
- Heavy Metal Support by Thorne—replaces important minerals and other nutrients lost during metal chelating
- Toxic Relief Booster by Thorne—nutrients designed to aid in metabolizing the increased amount of fat-stored toxins released into the bloodstream during a cleanse
- Formaldehyde Relief by Thorne—provides nutrients necessary for detoxification of formaldehyde from new carpet and furniture outgassing, as well as compounds produced by *Candida albicans* or by alcohol metabolism
- Solvent Remover by Thorne—contains amino acids specific to solvent detoxification in the liver, as well as nutrients that help protect nerves from solvent damage
- Pesticide Protector by Thorne—aids in detoxification of chlorinated pesticides, organophosphates, carbamates, and pyrethrins

INFORMATION AND PRODUCTS FOR SPECIFIC DISORDERS

Sleep disorders and the amino acid program
Testing neurotransmitters is the best way to determine if you have depletion in brain chemicals. Testing can be completed whether you are taking medications or not. You can determine if your neurotransmitters are out of balance by taking the Brain Wellness Program's Self Test. Just go to www.Neurogistics.com and click "Get Started." Use the practitioner code SLEEP (all caps). You can order

the program, which includes a urine in-home test that will yield a report on your neurotransmitter levels. You'll be given a customized protocol with guidelines for the right amino acids for you to take to help correct your imbalances. Or you can call 866.843.8935 for more information.

Appendix B

Health Centers Utilizing Juice and Raw Foods Cleanse Programs

HE FOLLOWING CENTERS offer a raw foods and/or juice detoxification program. Most of them offer nutritional classes, and some offer other health classes that address the emotional, mental, and spiritual aspects of health and renewal. Most of the centers also offer massage and colonics. It is best to contact the various centers to find out which one best fits your needs.

Cedar Springs Renewal Center
Michael Mahaffey and Nan Monk, Directors
31459 Barben Road
Sedro Woolley, WA 98284
Phone: 360.826.3599
Fax: 360.422.1524
Web site: www.cedarsprings.org

HealthQuarters Ministries
David Frahm, ND, Director
3620 W. Colorado Ave.
Colorado Springs, CO 80904
Phone: 719.593.8694
Fax: 719.531.7884
E-mail: healthqu@healthquarters.org
Web site: www.healthquarters.org

Hippocrates Institute
Brian and Anna Maria Clement, Directors
1443 Palmdale Ct.

West Palm Beach, FL 33411
Phone: 800.842.2125
Fax: 561.471.9464
E-mail: hippocrates@worldnet.att.net
Web site: www.hippocratesinstitute.org

Optimum Health Institute of Austin
Route 1 Box 339 J
Cedar Creek, TX 78612
Phone: 512.303.4817
Fax: 512.303.1239
E-mail: austin@optimumhealth.org
Web site: www.optimumhealth.org

Optimum Health Institute of San Diego
6970 Central Ave.
Lemon Grove, CA 91945-2198
Phone: 800.993.4325
Fax: 619.589.4098
E-mail: optimum@optimumhealth.org
Web site: www.optimumhealth.org

Sanoviv Medical Institute
Dr. Myron Wentz, Director
Playa de Rosarito, Km 39
Baja, California, Mexico
Phone: 800.726.6848
Fax: 801.954.7477
Web site: www.sanoviv.com

We Care
Susana and Susan Lombardi, Directors
18000 Long Canyon Rd.
Desert Hot Springs, CA 92241
Phone: 800.888.2523
Fax: 760.251.5399
E-mail: info@wecarespa.com
Web site: www.wecarespa.com

Notes

Chapter 1—The Turbo Diet

1. Megan Rauscher, "Vegetable Juice May Help With Weight Loss," Reuters.com, April 22, 2009, http://www.reuters.com/article/id USTRE53L60S20090422 (accessed February 5, 2010).

2. MedicalNewsToday.com, "Vegetable Use Aided in Dietary Support for Weight Loss and Lower Blood Pressure," October 21, 2009, http://www.medicalnewstoday.com/articles/168174.php (accessed February 5, 2010).

3. Ibid.

4. Ibid.

5. WebMD.com, "What Is Metabolic Syndrome?" January 25, 2009, http://www.webmd.com/heart/metabolic-syndrome/metabolic -syndrome-what-is-it (accessed January 27, 2010).

6. Ron Rosedale, "Insulin and Its Metabolic Effects," Mercola .com, July 14, 2001, http://articles.mercola.com/sites/articles/ archive/2001/07/14/insulin-part-one.aspx (accessed January 27, 2010).

7. Heather Basciano, Lisa Federico, and Khosrow Adeli, "Fructose, Insulin Resistance, and Metabolic Dyslipidemia," *Nutrition and Metabolism* 2, no. 5 (2005): http://www.nutritionandmetabolism .com/content/2/1/5 (accessed February 5, 2010).

8. Richard Fogoros, "Low Glycemic Weight Loss Is Longer Lasting," About.com: Heart Disease, http://heartdisease.about.com/od/ dietandobesity/a/logly.htm (accessed March 12, 2010).

9. Leslie Kenton and S. Kenton, *Raw Energy* (New York: Warner Books, 1986).

10. Jennie Brand-Miller, "A Glycemic Index Expert Responds to the Tufts Research," DiabetesHealth.com, October 18, 2007, http:// www.diabeteshealth.com/read/2007/10/18/5496/a-glycemic-index -expert-responds-to-the-tufts-research (accessed February 5, 2010).

Chapter 2—Juice Off the Pounds!

1. Jeannelle Boyer and Rui Hai Liu, "Apple Phytochemicals and Their Health Benefits," *Nutrition Journal* 3, no. 5 (May 2004), viewed at http://www.ncbi.nlm.nih.gov/pmc/articles/PMC442131/

(accessed January 27, 2010).

2. Hong Wang, Guohua Cao, and Ronald L. Prior, "Total Antioxidant Capacity of Fruits," *Journal of Agriculture and Food Chemistry* 44 (1996): 701–705, as viewed at http://ddr.nal.usda.gov/dspace/bitstream/10113/74/1/IND20626906.pdf (accessed January 27, 2010).

3. Renu Gandhi and Suzanne M. Snedeker, "Consumer Concerns About Pesticides in Food," Program on Breast Cancer and Environmental Risk Factors Fact Sheet #24, Cornell University, March 1999, http://envirocancer.cornell.edu/FactSheet/Pesticide/fs24.consumer.cfm (accessed February 5, 2010).

4. D. Winchester, J. Huskins, and J. Ying, "Agrichemicals in Surface Water and Birth Defects in the United States," *Acta Paediatrica (Oslo, Norway)* 98, no. 4 (1992): 664–669.

5. A. Ascherio, H. Chen, M. G. Weisskopf, et al., "Pesticide Exposure and Risk for Parkinson's Disease," *Annals of Neurology* 60, no. 2 (2006): 197–203.

6. L. A. McCauley, W. K. Anger, M. Keifer, R. Langley, M. G. Robson, and D. Rohlman, "Studying Health Outcomes in Farmworker Populations Exposed to Pesticides," *Environmental Health Perspectives* 114, no. 3 (2006): 953–960.

7. TimesOnline.co.uk, "Official: Organic Really Is Better," October 28, 2007, http://www.timesonline.co.uk/tol/news/uk/health/article2753446.ece (accessed January 28, 2010).

8. Virginia Worthington, "Nutritional Quality of Organic Versus Conventional Fruits, Vegetables, and Grains," *Journal of Alternative and Complementary Medicine* 7, no. 2 (2001): 161–173, as viewed at http://www.ioia.net/images/pdf/orgvalue.pdf (accessed January 28, 2010).

9. Tara Parker-Pope, "Five Easy Ways to Go Organic," *New York Times*, October 22, 2007, http://well.blogs.nytimes.com/2007/10/22/five-easy-ways-to-go-organic/ (accessed January 28, 2010).

10. Ibid.

11. Bob Williams, "Produce Treated With Pesticides Not Limited to Grocery Stores," *Fergus Falls Journal*, August 8, 2007, http://www.ewg.org/node/22379 (accessed January 28, 2010).

12. Environmental Working Group, "The Full List: 47 Fruits and Veggies," Shopper's Guide to Pesticides, http://www.foodnews.org/fulllist.php (accessed January 28, 2010).

13. George L. Tritsch, quoted in TrueHealth.org, "'Nuked Food'—

the Dangers of Irradiated Food," http://www.truehealth
.org/nukedfood.html (accessed February 5, 2010).

14. G. Löfroth, "Toxic Effects of Irradiated Foods," *Nature* 211 (July
16, 1966): 302, abstract viewed at http://www.nature.com/nature/
journal/v211/n5046/pdf/211302a0.pdf (accessed February 5, 2010).

15. J. S. de Vendômois, F. Roullier, D. Cellier, and G. E. Séralini,
"A Comparison of the Effects of Three GM Corn Varieties on
Mammalian Health," *International Journal of Biological Sciences*
5 (2009): 706–726, http://www.biolsci.org/v05p0706.htm (accessed
February 5, 2010).

16. David Derbyshire, "Fears Grow as Study Shows Genetically
Modified Crops 'Can Cause Liver and Kidney Damage,'"
DailyMail.co.uk, January 21, 2010, http://www.dailymail.co.uk
/news/article-1244824/Fears-grow-study-shows-genetically-
modified-crops-cause-liver-kidney-damage.html (accessed February
5, 2010).

17. de Vendômois, Roullier, Cellier, and Séralini, "A Comparison of
the Effects of Three GM Corn Varieties on Mammalian Health."

18. James E. McWilliams, "The Green Monster," Slate.com, January
28, 2009, http://www.slate.com/id/2209168/pagenum/all/ (accessed
February 8, 2010).

19. "Regulation of Foods Derived From Plants," statement of Lester
M. Crawford before the Subcommittee on Conservation, Rural
Development, and Research House Committee on Agriculture,
June 17, 2003, http://www.fda.gov/NewsEvents/Testimony/
ucm161037.htm (accessed February 8, 2010).

20. Deborah B. Whitman, "Genetically Modified Foods: Harmful
or Helpful?" CSA Discovery Guide, April 2000, http://www.csa
.com/discoveryguides/gmfood/overview.php (accessed February 8,
2010).

21. Ibid., referencing Jorge Fernandez-Cornejo and William D.
McBride, "Genetically Engineered Crops for Pest Management,"
Agricultural Economic Report No. 786, April 2000, http://www
.ers.usda.gov/publications/aer786/aer786.pdf (accessed February 8,
2010).

22. Emma Young, "GM Pea Causes Allergic Damage in Mice,"
NewScientist.com, November 21, 2005, http://www.newscientist
.com/article/dn8347 (accessed February 8, 2010).

23. Mavis Butcher, "Genetically Modified Food—GM Foods List
and Information," Disabled-World.com, September 22, 2009,

http://www.disabled-world.com/fitness/gm-foods.php   (accessed February 8, 2010).

CHAPTER 3—THE ALKALINIZING BENEFITS OF THE TURBO DIET

1. A. Milosevic, "Sports Drinks Hazard to Teeth," *British Journal of Sports Medicine* 31, issue 1 (1997): 28–30, abstract viewed at http://bjsm.bmj.com/content/31/1/28.abstract (accessed January 28, 2010).

2. Robert O. Young and Shelley Radford Young, *The pH Miracle for Weight Loss* (New York: Warner Books, 2006).

3. Ute Alexy, Mathilde Kersting, and Thomas Remer, "Potential Renal Acid Load in the Diet of Children and Adolescents: Impact of Food Groups, Age and Time Trends," *Public Health Nutrition* 11, no. 3 (July 5, 2007): 300–306, viewed at http://journals.cambridge .org/action/displayFulltext?type=1&fid=1700856&jid=PHN&volu meId=11&issueId=03&aid=1700848 (accessed January 28, 2010).

4. NobelPrize.org, "Physiology of Digestion," Ivan Pavlov Nobel Lecture, December 12, 1904, http://nobelprize.org/nobel_prizes/ medicine/laureates/1904/pavlov-lecture.html (accessed January 29, 2010).

5. William Howard Hay, *Health Via Food*, tenth edition (n.p.: Sun-Health Diet Foundation, 1933); William Howard Hay, *Weight Control* (n.p.: Hay System, 1935); James Khan, "Does an Alkaline Diet Help You Lose Weight? A Review of the Evidence," Ezinearticles.com, January 28, 2006, http://ezinearticles .com/?Does-An-Alkaline-Diet-Help-You-Lose-Weight?-A-Review -Of-The-Evidence&id=135719 (accessed February 8, 2010).

6. F. Garcia-Contreras, R. Paniagua, M. Avila-Diaz, et al., "Cola Beverage Consumption Induces Bone Mineralization Reduction in Ovariectomized Rats," *Archives of Medical Research* 31, no 4 (July–August 2000): 360–365, abstract viewed at http://www.ncbi .nlm.nih.gov/pubmed/11068076 (accessed January 28, 2010).

7. B. Dawson-Hughes, S. S. Harris, and L. Ceglia, "Alkaline Diets Favor Lean Tissue Mass in Older Adults," *American Journal of Clinical Nutrition* 87, no. 3 (March 2008): 662–665.

8. L. Frassetto, R. C. Morris Jr., D. E. Sellmeyer, K. Todd, and A. Sebastian, "Diet, Evolution, and Aging—the Pathophysiologic Effects of the Post-Agricultural Inversion of the Potassium-to-Sodium and Base-to-Chloride Ratios in the Human Diet," *European Journal of Nutrition* 40, no. 5 (October 2001): 200–213, abstract viewed at http://www.ncbi.nlm.nih.gov/pubmed/11842945

(accessed January 29, 2010).

9. H. M. Macdonald, S. A. New, W. D. Frase, M. K. Campbell, and D. M. Reid, "Low Dietary Potassium Intakes and High Dietary Estimates of Net Endogenous Acid Production Are Associated With Low Bone Mineral Density in Premenopausal Women and Increased Markers of Bone Resorption in Postmenopausal Women," *American Journal of Clinical Nutrition* 81, no. 4 (April 2005): 923–933.

10. S. T. Reddy, C. Y. Wang, K. Sakhaee, L. Brinkley, and C. Y. Pak, "Effect of Low-Carbohydrate High-Protein Diets on Acid-Base Balance, Stone-Forming Propensity, and Calcium Metabolism," *American Journal of Kidney Disease* 40, no. 2 (August 2002): 265–274.

11. Sang Y. Whang, *Reverse Aging* (Miami: JSP Publishing, 1991).

CHAPTER 4—THE TURBO DIET EXERCISE PLAN

1. Sharon Howard, "Diet and Strength Training," ESPN Training Room, http://www.espn.go.com/trainingroom/s/2000/0225/380656.html (accessed January 29, 2010).

CHAPTER 5—TROUBLESHOOTING: WHAT TO
DO WHEN YOU DON'T LOSE WEIGHT

1. A conversation Dr. Robert C. Atkins had with Brenda Watson, author of *Gut Solutions*, as related to Cherie Calbom by Brenda Watson, February 2004.

2. Susan E. Swithers and Terry L. Davidson, "A Role for Sweet Taste: Calorie Predictive Relations in Energy Regulation by Rats," *Behavioral Neuroscience* 122, no. 1 (February 2008): 161–173, abstract viewed at http://psycnet.apa.org/journals/bne/122/1/161/ (accessed January 29, 2010).

3. J. H. Lavin, S. J. French, and N. W. Read, "The Effect of Sucrose- and Aspartame-Sweetened Drinks on Energy Intake, Hunger, and Food Choice of Female, Moderately Restrained Eaters," *International Journal of Obesity* 21, no. 1 (January 1997): 37–42, viewed at http://www.nature.com/ijo/journal/v21/n1/pdf/0800360a.pdf (accessed January 29, 2010).

4. 65th Annual Scientific Sessions of the American Diabetes Association, June 10–14, 2005, San Diego, CA, Abstract 1085-P, as quoted in "Aspartame and Weight Gain," HolisticMed.com, http://www.holisticmed.com/aspartame/recent.html (accessed February 8, 2010).

5. M. B. Abou-Donia, E. M. El-Masry, A. A. Abdel-Rahman, R. E. McLendon, and S. S. Schiffman, "Splenda Alters Gut Microflora and Increases Intestinal p-Glycoprotein and Cytochrome p-450 in Male Rats," *Journal of Toxicology and Environmental Health* 71, no. 21 (2008): 1415–1419, abstract viewed at http://www.ncbi.nlm .nih.gov/sites/entrez (accessed January 29, 2010).

6. Craig Lambert, "Deep Into Sleep," *Harvard Magazine*, July–August 2005, http://harvardmagazine.com/2005/07/deep-into-sleep.html (accessed January 29, 2010).

7. National Sleep Foundation, *2005 Sleep in America Poll*, March 29, 2005, http://www.sleepfoundation.org/sites/default/files/2005_ summary_of_findings.pdf (accessed January 29, 2010).

8. James E. Gangwisch, Dolores Malaspina, Bernadette Boden-Albala, and Steven B. Heymsfield, "Inadequate Sleep as a Risk Factor for Obesity: Analyses of the NHANES 1," *Sleep* 28, no. 10 (2005): 1289–1296, viewed at http://www .journalsleep.org/Articles/281017.pdf (accessed February 2, 2010).

9. Gudmundur Bergsson, Jóhann Arnfinnsson, Ólafur Steingrímsson, and Halldor Thormar, "In Vitro Killing of *Candida albicans* by Fatty Acids and Monoglycerides," *Antimicrobial Agents and Chemotherapy* 45, no. 11 (November 2001): 3209–3212, viewed at http://aac.asm.org/cgi/content/full/45/11/3209 (accessed February 2, 2010).

10. Ibid.

CHAPTER 6—EMOTIONAL EATING, BINGE
EATING, AND FOOD ADDICTIONS

1. Angela Stokes, *Raw Emotions* (Garden City, NY: Monarch Publishing, 2009).

2. Melinda Beck, "Putting an End to Mindless Munching," *Wall Street Journal*, May 13, 2008, http://online.wsj.com/article/ SB121062985377986351.html (accessed February 3, 2010).

CHAPTER 7—THE TURBO DIET PLAN

1. EatWild.com, "Summary of Important Health Benefits of Grassfed Meats, Eggs, and Dairy," http://www.eatwild.com/healthbenefits .htm (accessed February 3, 2010).

2. C. Ip, J. A. Scimeca, and H. J. Thompson, "Conjugated Linoleic Acid: A Powerful Anticarcinogen From Animal Fat Sources," *Cancer* 74, suppl. 3 (August 1, 1994): 1050–1054; K. L. Houseknecht, J. P. Vanden Heuvel, S. Y. Moya-Camarena, et al., "Dietary Conjugated

Linoleic Acid Normalizes Impaired Glucose Tolerance in the Zucker Diabetic Fatty Fa/Fa Rat," *Biochemical and Biophysical Research Communications* 244, no. 3 (March 27, 1998): 678–682, abstract viewed at http://www.ncbi.nlm.nih.gov/pubmed/9535724 (accessed February 3, 2010).

3. Randy Shaver, "By-Product Feedstuffs in Dairy Cattle Diets in the Upper Midwest," http://www.uwex.edu/ces/dairynutrition/documents/byproductfeedsrevised2008.pdf (accessed February 3, 2010).

4. G. C. Smith, "Dietary Supplementation of Vitamin E to Cattle to Improve Shelf Life and Case Life of Beef for Domestic and International Markets," Colorado State University, referenced in EatWild.com, "Summary of Important Health Benefits of Grassfed Meats, Eggs, and Dairy."

5. W. G. Kruggel, R. A. Field, G. J. Miller, K. M. Horton, and J. R. Busboom, "Influence of Sex and Diet on Lutein in Lamb Fat," *Journal of Animal Science* 54 (1982): 970–975, abstract viewed at http://jas.fass.org/cgi/content/abstract/54/5/970 (accessed February 3, 2010).

6. Dan Flynn, "Russia Bans U.S. Poultry Over Chlorine," *Food Safety News*, January 7, 2010, http://www.foodsafetynews.com/2010/01/russia-bans-us-poultry-over-chlorine/ (accessed February 3, 2010).

7. EatWild.com, "Summary of Important Health Benefits of Grassfed Meats, Eggs, and Dairy."

8. World-wire.com, "American Public Health Association Supports Ban on Hormonal Milk and Meat," news release, November 13, 2009, http://www.world-wire.com/news/0911130001.html (accessed February 8, 2010).

9. ConsumerReports.org. "Chicken: Arsenic and Antibiotics," July 2007, http://www.consumerreports.org/cro/food/food-safety/animal-feed-and-food/animal-feed-and-the-food-supply-105/chicken-arsenic-and-antibiotics/index.htm (accessed February 3, 2010).

10. Tabitha Alterman, "Eggciting News!" MotherEarthNews.com, October 15, 2008, http://www.motherearthnews.com/Relish/Pastured-Eggs-Vitamin-D-Content.aspx (accessed February 3, 2010).

11. Cheryl Long and Tabitha Alterman, "Meet Real Free-Range Eggs," MotherEarthNews.com, October/November 2007, http://www.motherearthnews.com/Real-Food/2007-10-01/Tests-Reveal

-Healthier-Eggs.aspx (accessed February 3, 2010).

12. Ibid.

13. S. E. Swithers and T. L. Davidson, "A Role for Sweet Taste: Calorie Predictive Relations in Energy Regulation by Rats," *Behavioral Neuroscience* 122, no. 1 (February 2008): 161–173, referenced in ScienceDaily.com, "Artificial Sweeteners Linked to Weight Gain," February 11, 2008, http://www.sciencedaily.com/releases/2008/02/080210183902.htm (accessed February 3, 2010).

14. U.S. Department of Agriculture, *Pesticide Data Program: Annual Summary Calendar Year 2005* (Washington: Agricultural Marketing Service, 2006), http://www.ams.usda.gov/AMSv1.0/getfile?dDocName=STELPRDC5049946 (accessed February 3, 2010).

15. Virginia Worthington, "Nutritional Quality of Organic Versus Conventional Fruits, Vegetables, and Grains," *Journal of Alternative and Complementary Medicine* 7, no 2 (April 2001): 161–173, abstract viewed at http://www.liebertonline.com/doi/abs/10.1089/107555301750164244 (accessed February 3, 2010).

16. Alice Park, "Can Sugar Substitutes Make You Fat?" *TIME*, February 10, 2008, http://www.time.com/time/health/article/0,8599,1711763,00.html (accessed February 4, 2010).

17. Woodrow C. Monte, "Aspartame: Methanol and Public Health," *Journal of Applied Nutrition* 36, no. 1 (1984): 44, referenced in documentary *Sweet Misery* (Tucson, AZ: Sound and Fury Productions, 2004), http://www.soundandfury.tv/pages/sweet%20misery.html (accessed February 4, 2010).

18. Ibid., also, Dani Veracity, "The Link Between Aspartame and Brain Tumors: What the FDA Never Told You About Artificial Sweeteners," NaturalNews.com, September 22, 2005, http://www.naturalnews.com/011804_aspartame_tumors_brain_tumor.html (accessed February 4, 2010).

19. Joanne Waldron, "Duke University Study Links Splenda to Weight Gain, Health Problems," NaturalNews.com, October 20, 2008, http://www.naturalnews.com/024543.html (accessed February 4, 2010).

20. Abou-Donia, El-Masry, Abdel-Rahman, McLendon, Schiffman, "Splenda Alters Gut Microflora and Increases Intestinal p-Glycoprotein and Cytochrome p-450 in Male Rats."

21. D. Benton and R. Cook, "Selenium Supplementation Improves Mood in a Double-Blind Crossover Trial," *Psychopharmacology* 102, no. 4 (1990): 549–550, abstract viewed at http://www.ncbi

.nlm.nih.gov/pubmed/2096413 (accessed February 4, 2010).

22. *International Journal of Obesity and Related Metabolic Disorders* (September 16, 2003), referenced in "Calcium and Weight Loss," In Focus Newsletter, May 2005, http://www.nutricology.com/In -Focus-Newsletter-May-2005-sp-45.html (accessed February 4, 2010).

23. Y. C. Lin, R. M. Lyle, L. D. McCabe, G. P. McCabe, C. M. Weaver, and D. Teegarden, "Daily Calcium Is Related to Changes in Body Composition During a Two-Year Exercise Intervention in Young Women," *Journal of the American College of Nutrition* 19, no 6 (November–December 2000): 754–760, abstract viewed at http:// www.ncbi.nlm.nih.gov/pubmed/11194528 (accessed February 4, 2010).

24. K. M. Davies, R. P. Heaney, R. R. Recker, et al., "Calcium Intake and Body Weight," *Journal of Clinical Endocrinology and Metabolism* 85, no. 12 (December 2000): 4635–4638, abstract viewed at http:// www.ncbi.nlm.nih.gov/pubmed/11134120 (accessed February 4, 2010).

25. *Endocrine Today*, "High Levels of Vitamin D, Low-Caloric Diet May Increase Weight Loss," December 31, 2009, http://www .endocrinetoday.com/view.aspx?rid=59663 (accessed February 4, 2010).

26. F. Ceci, C. Cangiano, M. Cairella, et al., "The Effects of Oral 5-Hydroxytryptophan Administration on Feeding Behavior in Obese Adult Female Subjects," *Journal of Neural Transmission* 76, no. 2 (1989): 109–117.

27. C. Cangiano, F. Ceci, M. Cairella, et al., "Effects of 5-Hydroxytryptophan on Eating Behavior and Adherence to Dietary Prescriptions in Obese Adult Subjects," *Advances in Experimental Medicine and Biology* 294 (1991): 591–593.

28. Steven A. Abrams, Ian J. Griffin, Keli M. Hawthorne, and Kenneth J. Ellis, "Effect of Prebiotic Supplementation and Calcium Intake on Body Mass Index," *Journal of Pediatrics* 151, no. 3 (September 2007): 293–298, abstract viewed at http://www.jpeds.com/article/ S0022-3476(07)00280-6/abstract (accessed February 4, 2010).

CHAPTER 9—THE TURBO DIET RECIPES

1. L. W. Blau, "Cherry Diet Control for Gout and Arthritis," *Texas Reports on Biology and Medicine* 8 (1950): 309–311.

Index

Home Juice Parties!

Find out how to start juice parties for weight loss and healthy living in your home, church, or organization. Facilitate juice parties that can change people's lives. From weight loss to healthy living, you can become a change agent in your community. For more information, call 866-843-8935.

Schedule Cherie to Speak for Your Organization

To schedule Cherie Calbom, MSN, to speak at your church, organization, or town as a keynote speaker or for other speaking engagements, workshops, and weekend retreats, call 866-843-8935.

Topics include:

- The Turbo Juice Weight Loss Program
- Juicing and Raw Foods for Vibrant Health
- Juice Fasting for Weight Loss and Improved Health
- Juicing and Raw Foods Demonstrations
- Letting Go of Emotional Eating with Fr. John and Cherie Calbom
- Emotional Freedom Through Emotional Cleansing Programs with Fr. John
- Achieving Vitality to Complete Your God-Given Purpose
- From Trials to Triumph: Cherie's Journey to Wholeness

Health and Weight Loss Coaching and Health Retreats

Fr. John and Cherie bring together an exciting and integrated spirit, soul, and body approach that encourage health, healing, and wholeness.

- Health and Weight Loss Coaching with Cherie Calbom, MSN, or Fr. John Calbom, MA (counseling psychology)
- Health Retreats: Lifestyle programs that include diet, juicing, fasting, and detoxing for healing, weight loss, and disease prevention.

For more information, call 866-843-8935.